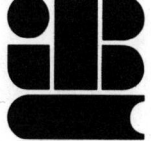

Consultation Skills for Health Care Professionals

Francis L. Ulschak
Sharon M. SnowAntle

Foreword by Nicolas C. Porter

Consultation Skills for Health Care Professionals

How to Be an Effective Consultant Within Your Organization

Jossey-Bass Publishers
San Francisco • Oxford • 1990

CONSULTATION SKILLS FOR HEALTH CARE PROFESSIONALS
How to Be an Effective Consultant Within Your Organization
by Francis L. Ulschak and Sharon M. SnowAntle

Copyright © 1990 by: Jossey-Bass Inc., Publishers
                              350 Sansome Street
                              San Francisco, California 94104
                              &
                              Jossey-Bass Limited
                              Headington Hill Hall
                              Oxford OX3 0BW

Copyright under International, Pan American, and Universal Copyright Conventions. All rights reserved. No part of this book may be reproduced in any form—except for brief quotation (not to exceed 1,000 words) in a review or professional work—without permission in writing from the publishers.

Library of Congress Cataloging-in-Publication Data

Ulschak, Francis L., date.
    Consultation skills for health care professionals : how to be an effective consultant within your organization / Francis L. Ulschak, Sharon M. SnowAntle ; foreword by Nicolas C. Porter. — 1st ed.
    p. cm. — (The Jossey-Bass health series)
    Includes bibliographical references (p.).
    ISBN 1-55542-239-X (alk. paper)
    1. Hospitals—Staff. 2. Medical consultation. 3. Interpersonal communication. I. SnowAntle, Sharon M., date. II. Title.
III. Series.
RA972.U47   1990
362.1'1'0684—dc20   90-4103
                                                                CIP

Manufactured in the United States of America

The paper in this book meets the guidelines for permanence and durability of the Committee on Production Guidelines for Book Longevity of the Council on Library Resources.

JACKET DESIGN BY WILLI BAUM

FIRST EDITION

Code 9041

The Jossey-Bass
Health Series

Contents

Foreword *Nicolas C. Porter*	xi
Preface	xv
The Authors	xxi
Part I: The Need for Internal Consulting	**1**
1. How Internal Consulting Can Increase Organizational Effectiveness	3
2. The Roles and Skills of Internal Consultants	27
Part II: The Process of Internal Consulting	**53**
3. The Eight Stages in Internal Consulting	55
4. Establishing an Effective Relationship with the Client	74
5. Collecting and Analyzing Information	99
6. Presenting the Data	129

7.	Taking Action and Evaluating the Results	144

Part III: Becoming an Effective Internal Consultant — **167**

8.	Understanding the Culture of the Organization	169
9.	Sharpening Four Essential Interpersonal Skills	193
10.	Ethical Issues and Common Pitfalls	228
11.	The Keys to Successful Internal Consulting	246
	References	251
	Index	255

Foreword

The pressures facing health care today are enormous. Government, business, and the public demand that the cost of hospital services be controlled or reduced. At the same time, the Joint Commission on the Accreditation of Healthcare Organizations (JCAHO) Agenda for Change means demonstrated quality. Today, as health care consumers, we expect that hospitals will provide the latest in technologies, with access for all. Yet in 1989, the Harris Poll reported that 85 percent of the U.S. public is dissatisfied with the way we deliver health care.

The environment in which we manage these pressures is one of the most complex for leaders of any organization. The diversification runs the gamut, from the sophistication of the critical care unit or genotyping lab to parking and security, which must ensure the peace of mind and convenience of patients and staff alike.

It is incumbent on health care professions to become more effective in bringing health care costs and delivery under control. *Consultation Skills for Health Care Professionals* is a book that can provide leaders of hospital management teams with tools to address such problems. Francis Ulschak and Sharon SnowAntle bring together their considerable experience in hospital organizational development to provide a model for internal consulting in the health care industry. This model is designed to enhance the effectiveness of personnel in working together to achieve organizational goals.

Hospitals, for the most part, have been departmentalized. To be sure, the patient is the focal point of the various hospital departments. But each department's institutional focus becomes clouded by its internal requirements and specialization. Departments have "turfs."

The largest portion of any hospital's expenses is its employees. Employees are also the institution's most valuable asset. A tremendous wealth of expertise exists among a hospital's staff. Today, more than ever, we must rely on our internal expertise, which many times goes untapped or is overlooked in favor of outside services.

The internal consulting model provides a method for hospitals not only to improve costs and/or services but also to foster collaboration and cooperation. The model presented in this book provides instances in which the consulting process guides implementation across the diversities of the hospital environment. Out of these interactions grows a more effective and productive organization.

The information in the model is applicable whether your background is that of a physician or pharmacist, administrator or information systems analyst. As managers, directors, and leaders, we are responsible and accountable for accomplishing the goals and objectives of our organizations. The internal consulting model lends itself to implementing plans that support our objectives and also allows for the evaluation of the success of the internal consulting effort. In some ways, it is the evaluation step that differentiates internal consulting from external consulting. The model can be incorporated as part of the management accountability fabric of the organization. This will help ensure that the final outcome of the consultation process is not just a report.

Within academic institutions, the internal consulting model can be effective in dealing with the complexities of a tertiary health care facility in a university setting. The missions of service, education, and clinical and basic research can be in conflict. These missions also can be constrained by the pressures brought by health care reimbursement and cuts in government funding of education and research. The helping rela-

Foreword

tionships within the internal consulting model assist in managing these pressures and resolving these conflicts. The result is a more effective health care team.

Consultation Skills for Health Care Professionals could not be more timely. But we are not just concerned with the hurdles of today. AIDS, the aging population, a biohazardous environment, and many other challenges await us throughout the 1990s and into the next century. By making the internal consulting model part of your organization, you will be that much more secure in meeting the challenges to come.

Tampa, Florida Nicolas C. Porter
March 1990 *Executive Director*
 H. Lee Moffitt Cancer Center
 and Research Institute

Preface

The purpose of this book is simple—it is designed to increase the effectiveness of health care personnel in consulting with one another for the purpose of enhancing departmental or organizational effectiveness. Why is this important? Think for a moment about health care costs. For the year 1987, $500 billion were spent in health care. This represents 11 percent of the gross national product (State of Florida Health Care Cost Containment Board, 1988), and health care costs continue to rise.

Think for a moment about health care organizations. They are labor-intensive organizations filled with high-tech individuals. According to the Bureau of Labor Statistics (1987), there were 8,061,000 workers employed in the health care industry in 1986. This represents 7 percent of the labor force. A 40 percent increase (to 11,276,000) was projected for the year 2000 (Bureau of Labor Statistics, 1987). Those health care workers are skilled in the technical side but not necessarily the consultation side of their work. Health care organizations are highly dependent on these individuals' working together and consulting with each other. That is what this book is about.

Our belief is that the internal consulting skills model we are presenting for health care professionals will be an important key in increasing the working skills between health care professionals. We believe that the more effective these consulting skills are, the more effective will be the health care organization. And, as the Joint Commission on Accreditation of Hospital Organizations continues to look to the organization as the ultimate key in quality patient care, these skills increase in importance.

Audience

This book has several audiences. The first audience is those support groups within the health care organization that have a responsibility to assist the direct patient care team. These include the departments of human resources, education and training, marketing and planning, public relations, business, environmental services, volunteers, and others. These departments work with other departments in providing quality patient care.

The second audience is the direct patient care givers. This group includes nurses; physicians; social workers; laboratory, radiology, dietary, and respiratory technicians; and others. These care givers have direct interactions with others, and quality patient care will ultimately depend on the effectiveness of those interactions.

The third audience is the administration. Administration in health care organizations depends totally on others to do the work that leads to quality care. The model for internal consulting that we present and discuss is one administrators will find useful for getting the work done.

Benefits

What is the benefit of this book? Simply put, the benefit is a more effective health care team. Internal consulting defines an effective helping relationship that leads to effective outcomes. That effective helping relationship is the core of an effective health care team. Teams for us are project teams, for example, for information systems conversions, opening new units, closing down units, and the like.

There are other benefits of this book. Individuals in health care organizations may use it to evaluate their internal consulting skill level. The organization may want to use the book to develop training programs for key individuals whose

Preface

roles cause them to interact significantly with others. In fact, it was because of such a training program that we initially decided to write this book.

Overview

Our goal in this book is to present a model for internal consulting in health care organizations that will lead to effective consultations between and within departments. The book is divided into three sections.

Part One contains Chapters One and Two. The purpose of Part One is to lay the groundwork for internal consulting in health care organizations. It provides an introduction to the book and our beliefs regarding internal consulting.

Chapter One discusses the health care challenge in today's world. We define and discuss the role of the internal consultant in general and the internal consultant's relationship to the external consultant. A key theme is that the world of health care is in continuous and turbulent change. The internal consultant can be a useful model for operating in that system of change.

Chapter Two identifies the various roles of the internal consultant and the skills that go along with the roles. One unique aspect of this chapter is use of a model for assisting the health care profession in deciding the most useful internal consultant role to take in a particular consultation.

Part Two consists of Chapters Three through Seven. It goes into the actual process of internal consulting and outlines the eight steps of the consulting process.

Chapter Three discusses the fact that internal consulting is a process, not a single interaction with a client. This chapter overviews our view of that process. The chapter's purpose is to provide the reader with a "road map" of Chapters Four through Seven.

Our internal consulting process is an eight-stage process with decisions the internal consultant makes as he or she proceeds. Chapter Three closes with two case studies that walk through the model.

Chapter Four covers establishing an effective client relationship. A critical question for the internal consultant is "Who is my client?" Is it the person with whom the internal consultant is working? That person's manager? The consultant's manager? Chapter Four sorts out how to determine who the client is and how to define the effective consultant-client relationship.

Chapter Four introduces a model, which we call the CPR + F model, that we use throughout the remainder of the book. This model is an effective tool for reviewing the consultant-client relationship. Examples and pitfalls of contracting are discussed. Chapter Four, Chapters Five through Seven, and Chapters Nine and Ten contain skill questionnaires for internal consultant skills.

Chapter Five covers data collection and analysis. Almost every consultation involves collecting data of some type. The goal of Chapter Five is to provide tools for collecting data and analyzing it—that is, making sense of it. The chapter reviews the standard methods of data collection and provides examples of each and then provides hints on how to analyze the data collected.

In the internal consultant process, there comes a time when the findings from data collection are presented. This is the topic of Chapter Six. That data presentation may be to one person or to a group of persons. It may be informal or formal. Chapter Six explores this step of data presentation and provides the reader with hints regarding it.

Chapter Seven covers taking action and evaluation. Once the communication of findings has been accomplished, the next step is the development of action plans. In this step developing action plans, including the costing out of various options, are explored. The action plan has the components of what is to be done, by whom, by what date, and with what resources.

Chapter Seven concludes with a discussion of evaluation. In evaluation the question "Did we get done what we needed to in a resource-efficient manner?" is finally asked.

Another topic in Chapter Seven is the termination of the consulting relationship. Again, we define the internal consultant role as a helping relationship that has an organizational or

Preface

departmental outcome attached to it. This means that we need to look at results as well as what it means to terminate the relationship.

Part Three contains Chapters Eight through Eleven. It is concerned with understanding some of the key variables surrounding internal consulting. Internal consulting happens in an environment of an organization. There are specific generic skills needed for internal consulting to happen. Part Three deals with these issues.

Internal consulting does not happen in a vacuum; it happens in the culture of an organization. Chapter Eight discusses the culture of an organization and how the internal consultant needs to take that culture into consideration in using the consulting process we have discussed.

One aspect of organizational culture is the organization's life cycle. Where the organization is at in its life cycle will impact how the consultation will be lived out.

For each step in the consultation process, we identify specific skills that were needed for that step. However, there are several basic skills needed for effective internal consulting. Four that we identify and discuss in Chapter Nine are listening skills, influence skills, conflict management skills, and problem-solving skills. The chapter closes with a complete skills checklist for the internal consultant.

Throughout the book we discuss the internal consultant role and how it is an important helper-helpee relationship. Many issues arise in the consultation that we consider to be ethical issues. Chapter Ten explores in detail some of the common pitfalls and what to do to avoid them.

The beginning of Chapter Eleven is a summary of the key learnings from Chapters One through Ten. We want to provide you with what we consider to be the most important statements. We also discuss resources in this chapter. What is needed to obtain the skills we have been discussing? What resources, human and material, are around that can assist the internal consultant? We provide several ideas about where the internal consultant can turn for additional training and assistance.

One last comment. Our ideal with this book would be to

discuss the concepts and ideas with you face to face. Unfortunately, that is not feasible. The next best option is to provide you with many opportunities throughout the book to dialogue with us. We have provided numerous exercises so that you might better understand the process we are describing. In that way, this book is interactive. We encourage you to make notes throughout. Make this a useful book experience for yourself.

Acknowledgments

A book like this does not happen solely because of those whose names are on the cover. First and foremost are all the individuals who let us work with them over the years. Because they were willing to have us work in their departments, we were able to gather the experiences necessary to write this book. In addition, there are several people we want to acknowledge. Judy Pins, Tricia Stream, and Linda Hunter took time to critique our early draft of this book, and their comments were useful for us. Cody Northrup has spent many hours reviewing the drafts and making editorial comments. Also important for us are our families. Writing this book meant long hours of work that at times conflicted with family time. We express our appreciation for the patience our families have shown.

Tampa, Florida Francis L. Ulschak
March 1990 Sharon M. SnowAntle

The Authors

Francis L. Ulschak is the assistant administrator for strategic resources at the H. Lee Moffitt Cancer Center and Research Institute, Tampa, Florida. He has a B.S. degree (1966) from Dickinson State College, an M.Div. degree (1970) from Garrett Theological Seminary, a Ph.D. degree (1975) from Northwestern University, and a master's of human resource development degree (1982) from University Associates.

Ulschak has worked extensively in the area of training and development in health care organizations. His major area of interest is team development and conflict management. He has received the American Society for Health Care Education and Training's Distinguished Service Award (1989) and Distinguished Achievement Award (1986).

Ulschak's other books include *Small Group Problem Solving: An Aid to Organizational Effectiveness* (1981), *Human Resource Development: The Theory and Practice of Needs Assessment* (1983), *Team Building in the Operating Room* (1989), and *Creating the Future of Healthcare Education* (1988).

Sharon M. SnowAntle is the director of education and organizational development at the H. Lee Moffitt Cancer Center and Research Institute, Tampa, Florida. She has a B. S. degree in nursing from Memorial University in Newfoundland, an M.S. degree in nursing from Boston University, and a Ph.D. degree from the University of South Florida.

SnowAntle has authored and coauthored articles in the areas of employee turnover, professional image, and health care trends. Her most recent publication on turnover prediction was in *Personnel Administrator* (June 1989).

Consultation Skills for Health Care Professionals

I

The Need for Internal Consulting

1

How Internal Consulting Can Increase Organizational Effectiveness

Imagine the following scenes:

You are an information resources person with responsibilities for working with departments to meet their information resource needs. Technically, you are very competent, yet you find that you frequently "miss the boat" with a department with which you are working. Your technical skills are intact. However, the skills you need to sit with another individual or department and to identify clearly what they need are weak. The result is that you find yourself spinning your wheels, which leads to frustration and ineffectiveness. When you come back to the client with what you thought they wanted, they report that they really wanted something else. The client group is not satisfied with your work, and neither are you.

You are in the lab and are working with a nursing department regarding the delivery of lab services. Again, your technical skills as a lab technician are excellent. However, there seem to be ongoing misunderstandings between you and the nursing group. They report that their needs are left unidentified and unfulfilled. They are dissatisfied with the lab. It seems that the misunderstandings stem from the discussions regarding who will be doing what and when and what the final outcomes need to look like.

The above examples are what this book is all about. Our basic thesis is simple: health care organizations are high-tech, highly interdependent, people-intensive organizations. There are very highly skilled individuals who are dependent on other highly skilled individuals to get their job done. Quality patient care is the result of a team of individuals working together. This means that the more effective individuals are in working with one another, the more potential for effectiveness the organization has.

In this high-tech environment, the emphasis in the recruitment and selection process is on hiring the individual with excellent technical skills. Frequently, the emphasis is not on the individual's ability to work with others in interdepartmental teams or to negotiate differences with others, yet these abilities are as critical as technical skills in the health care environment.

We believe that technical skills alone are not sufficient for the health care organization of today to function effectively and efficiently. Today's health care professional also needs interpersonal skills that go beyond the technical. We are not talking about simple verbal and written communication skills. We are talking about a specific set of skills that we call internal consulting skills. These include basic abilities to communicate effectively both verbally and nonverbally. In addition, we associate specific skills with determining the need of the client (the individual or department with which you are working), identifying what role you will play in relation to that department, agreeing on what steps need to happen, and carrying out those steps.

Why are internal consulting skills valuable for organizational productivity and efficiency? Again, think for a moment about the typical health care organization. It is labor intensive. Sixty percent of the operating budget goes to human resources. If we are interested in increasing organizational effectiveness, we need to be concerned with the productivity of the departments and individuals involved. Increasing the effectiveness of internal consulting, which happens naturally within the organization, increases the effectiveness of the total organization.

Think for a moment about this example. A nursing unit approaches the audiovisual department with a request for a video to be made. The video is to identify key preoperative steps for surgery patients. The audiovisual personnel take on the project and begin to work with it in earnest. When they take the video back to the department manager for review, however, the department manager is upset with the video. She feels that it has missed the point. The result is that the video goes back to the audiovisual department for rework.

For us this is a good example of something that can happen very frequently in health care organizations. What happened? Because a specific consulting process was not walked through with the department, a key decision maker was missed. The result was rework. As a bottom line, that means decreased productivity and enhanced costs.

Another point we made earlier is that departments in the health care setting are dramatically interdependent. Within the health care institution are highly professional workers who depend on one another to get their jobs done. They may or may not have an appreciation for how skilled their colleagues are, but they know they have to work together for achievement of common goals. A key focus for increasing productivity and performance at the individual, departmental, and organizational levels is creating effective transfer of information between professionals in their own and other departments. That is where internal consulting comes in.

Internal consulting is designed to assist the individuals who have to walk the interface between departments. Consider one of the opening scenarios. If the information resources person does not accurately assess a client's needs, the result is any one (or all) of the following:

- Waste of time of the department with which the information resources person was working.
- Waste of the information resources person's time.

Figure 1. Blending Technical and Internal Consulting Skills.

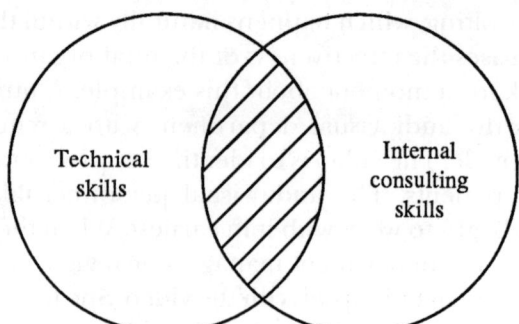

- Purchase of inappropriate hardware or software.
- Continued problems on the part of the department, possibly resulting in lost charges and the like.
- Failure to meet an organizational need.
- Ineffectiveness within the department.
- Ineffectiveness of mission for the health care organization. For most of us, this mission has to do with service to patients and their families.
- Others. Take a moment and think about others that you would add to this list.

If the information resources person had possessed good internal consulting skills—the skills with which this book is designed to assist—there would probably have been accurate contracting with the department regarding their needs. Next, an action plan would have been put together. The action plan would have been implemented and the outcomes evaluated. Hopefully, the end result would have been a problem that was "history."

The effective health care professional of the 1990s will blend the technical skills of her or his own profession and the internal consulting skills presented in this book. The model for internal consulting that we use throughout this book is illustrated in Figure 1.

The internal consultant has a balance between technical

How Internal Consulting Can Increase Effectiveness 7

skills and internal consulting skills. The next chapters will identify in detail the roles that the internal consultant will play along with the needed skills.

Who Is the Internal Consultant?

Take a moment and think of the associations that you have with the word *consultant*. When you hear the term, what comes to your mind?

Most of the time, when this question is asked, people report "good news" or "bad news." The "bad news" includes comments like:

> "The consultant is a person who is trying to get me to buy his wares."
> "The consultant is someone who is more than a hundred miles from home."
> "The consultant will sell me and leave me."
> "The consultant is someone who could not do anything else, so he became a consultant."

There is also the "good news":

> "The consultant is the person who saved me from certain destruction by getting me the information I needed."
> "The consultant is the person I was able to hire temporarily to help me through a crunch."
> "The consultant is an expert whom I can access but cannot afford to hire."

Our workshop experience tells us that people do have images about consultants that are important to identify and discuss.

One of the questions that is probably in your mind is: Who exactly is the internal consultant? The internal consultant is an individual who brings either technical expertise or process expertise to a setting. The dictionary defines a consultant as one who gives to another technical or professional advice. This definition has its core in the word *consult*, which means to call together, as in a senate, and ask for advice. To consult means "to seek information or instruction from."

The internal consultant, then, is one who consults with others to provide needed information and/or instruction. There are two parts to this. First, the consultant needs to have the knowledge, skills, or wisdom that another person or department needs or the ability to access that knowledge and those skills. Second, the consultant also needs to have skills in "fleshing out" what the department really needs. What are the real issues here? A standard assumption in internal consulting is that the presenting problem is rarely the real issue but rather is often just a symptom. As with a medical diagnosis, other information is needed. The consultant who simply takes a client's statement at face value may be missing the boat. The internal consultant needs to be a detective who goes about uncovering the facts relating to a problem.

The role of the internal consultant, then, is to help the client think through what the problem is (or how to arrive at what the problem is) and then to assist the client in resolving the problem.

The internal consultant is a giver of expert advice. "Expert advice" is a noble and dangerous gift. There is the story of a grade school student who was asked if she knew who Socrates was. Her response was: "Socrates was a very wise man who gave people good advice. So they poisoned him."

For internal consultants working with a variety of departments, there is an element of truth in this response. It is important to be sensitive to the advice you are giving.

Departments Involved in Internal Consulting

Our thesis is that the internal consultant role is vital for individuals in the health care organization who need to work the interface between departments. This applies to most departments in health care settings (see Figure 2).

What are some of the departments or groups to which this

How Internal Consulting Can Increase Effectiveness 9

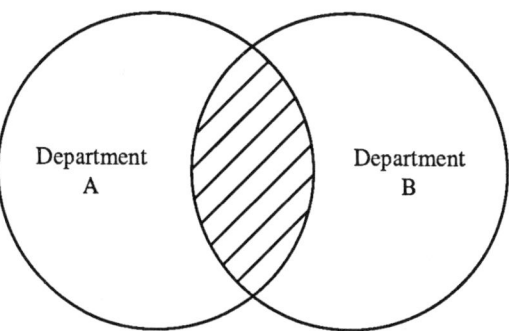

Figure 2. Interface Between Departments.

might apply? The following are some groups that we have identified in our experience in health care organizations.

Information Resources. Our opening scenario identifies individuals working in information resources as candidates for training in internal consultant skills. This is specially true when there is a conversion to a new system or significant training in the current system. The information resources person relates in significant ways to other departments in both giving and receiving of information. The clearer the definition of roles and expectations, the more effective the information resources person's work can be.

Education and Training. Education and training are a major ripe area when it comes to internal consultation. The education person spends a good deal of his or her time consulting with other departments on what their needs are and how to most effectively address those needs. In education it is easy to find costly examples of what happens when consulting skills break down or are not used. For instance, a health care educator might decide on an inappropriate training program because he or she failed to adequately contract with the client about what was needed. Ineffectiveness occurs when a training solution is offered to a nontraining problem. Significant losses in time and dollars can also occur, however, when segments of the health care organization are trained inappropriately or inadequately.

Human Resources. Human resources (HR) departments (or personnel) typically spend considerable time in consultation with other departments trying to identify or meet needs. Think about the process of recruitment and selection, for example. If the human resources person has not accurately assessed with the department manager the needs of a specific position, the result can be significant organizational energies expended in the recruitment of an individual who does not fit the job or the organizational culture.

The work of human resources primarily happens in consultation with other departments. Internal consulting skills apply to the areas of recruitment and selection, disciplinary actions, performance reviews, compensation plans, equal employment opportunity considerations, exit interviews, and human resources planning. If the human resources person is not skilled in internal consulting skills, the results can be very costly for the organization.

Hackett (1988, p. 70) states, "In many capacities, whether they are conscious of the fact, personnel executives are consultants—internal consultants—who need to possess and develop a unique set of behavioral as well as technical skills." This internal consultant role happens informally when the chief executive officer (CEO) or others ask the HR administrator for advice. Peters and Mabry (1981, p. 29) suggest that the internal consultant role replaces the adversarial role that frequently gets played out by the "personnel department." When the HR administrator is in the internal consultant role, she or he is considering the total organization and not just functions specific to her or his department. In such a case HR takes on a service approach, viewing the rest of the organization as a client system.

Lab, Radiology, Pharmacy, and Other Ancillary. The ancillary departments interface with all medical services within the health care organization. The goal is to have highly competent individuals. Each of these departments has its own internal

How Internal Consulting Can Increase Effectiveness 11

functioning and also has a critical interface with other departments. To do their work effectively, these departments need to monitor closely other departments and their needs. This means that the consultation skills again become useful.

Pastoral Care and Psychosocial Medicine. This is another group, frequently overlooked, for which internal consulting skills are critical. Typically, individuals who provide pastoral or psychosocial care are free to roam the entire health care facility. This means that they find themselves in situations where not only their professional expertise but also their consulting skills are sought. The chaplain is a good example. Frequently he or she responds to requests for assistance relating to employee or organizational issues. A manager may ask, "How should I go about handling this.... What should I do in that setting?" This group can be a significant force in resolving organizational blocks and increasing organizational effectiveness and efficiency.

Public Relations and Marketing. Public relations (PR) and marketing can benefit greatly from the skills of the internal consultant. In fact, much of PR and marketing has to do with negotiating with others. There is the PR item that has to be carefully developed with the client's needs in mind. Before the PR piece can be developed, there must be significant discussion with the client concerning what is needed. Consider, for example, a PR department developing a PR video for another department. If there is inappropriate identification of needs, the resulting video does not fit those needs. Good technical skills need to be enhanced by internal consultant skills.

Nursing. The largest single group in most health care organizations is the nursing department. Most hospitals need to be seen as nursing organizations. The reason people go to a hospital is that they are in need of specialized care that involves nursing services.

As the nurse acts as the patient's advocate, he or she

utilizes internal consulting skills on an hourly basis in interfacing with other departments.

Other departments and individuals could be added to the list. Two important criteria are:

1. The individual spends a good deal of his or her time in interfacing with other departments. Think about yourself for a moment. How much of your time is focused internally on your department, and how much is spent in working with other departments?

2. The work the individual does in other departments is in "servicing" that department. That means that the work is "client focused" with the other department being a client. If an individual works in significant ways with another department but his primary purpose is not to assist that department, he will not be doing internal consulting. For example, I may spend a lot of time working with HR in issues of recruitment for my staff. I am working with the HR department, but I am not consulting. Internal consulting means being engaged with that department to assist it with a problem it has identified.

This leads to the identification of another group that could benefit greatly from internal consultant skills—administration and management. Think for a moment about the discussion thus far. Key to the internal consultant role is that the individual is (1) working as the interface between his or her own department and another and (2) assisting the other department in the resolution of a problem.

Frequently, managers and administrators find themselves being asked by colleagues for assistance, in both formal and informal settings. The internal consultant model for the manager can be very useful in assisting other managers. In fact, the manager can use it as a way of building collegial and cooperative problem-solving ventures with other departments. The manager becomes "client centered." Internal consulting skills are vital for effectiveness. Our proposition: managers will find that internal consultant skills and ways of thinking can be a useful addition to their "skill bank."

We have one other comment regarding managers and internal consultant skills. Managers may find that internal con-

How Internal Consulting Can Increase Effectiveness

sultant skills are useful not only in dealing with other managers and directors but also in the management of their own departments. A manager who approaches her subordinates as an internal consultant will help them identify problems, find ways to resolve the problems, and keep clarity of roles. The result is that the manager will be able to get more work done through others by constantly raising the questions: What is it I can do to help you better get your job done? How can I be useful for you in getting the job done? The manager truly sees that her work gets done through assisting others to do their work more effectively.

To summarize, within health care institutions today, there are many groups that would find internal consulting skills to be an important addition. Many of these groups are already doing the work of internal consultants; they just might not be aware of it. The decision is whether to skill themselves with the needed resources to be more effective internal consultants.

Determining the Client

Throughout this book, we will use the term *client*. It is important to consider for a moment who the client is. Why? Without knowing who the client is, we will not be able to determine what we need to be about or what the final results need to be, and we are likely to end up in political battles. Whose needs are we meeting? Whose problem is needing resolution? It is like working in a department without knowing who your manager is or doing business with a firm and not dealing with the person who makes the decisions.

The client, using our definition, is the person who is the decision maker of the unit. He or she is the highest-level person in the department or organization who needs to be involved in the decision to have us work within that department or organization. He or she is the one who can implement what we propose and can have an immediate influence on the decision making.

To determine the client within the organization, the internal consultant needs to ask the following questions:

1. Is the person asking me to do this project in a position of authority to be asking? Does she or he have organizational

sanction to do the project? If the response is no, the person is not a client but is instead an interested party.

2. Is the person asking me to do this project able to implement the results of the project? Can he or she approve or disapprove it?

These questions help determine who the client is. However, our belief is that the ultimate client for the internal consultant in any organization is the organization itself. If the internal consultant runs into any problems, the question he or she must ask is: How does this impact the overall organization? This is a key difference between the external and the internal consultant. The external consultant may work for a department or a manager. The internal consultant always has the organizational interest in mind.

Trends Impacting Health Care

Why is the internal consultant role important? Our basic thesis is that having technically competent individuals skilled in internal consulting will increase organizational effectiveness. Their results will enhance the business side of the health care organization. Gone are the days of cost reimbursement in health care. This means that health care organizations will continue to be concerned with how to do things more effectively with less and will continue to "trim the fat" and juggle priorities.

Our point is that skilling current individuals in internal consulting will result in increased organizational effectiveness. Our formula is simple: (1) *technical skills combined with internal consulting skills lead to effective problem identification and resolution,* and (2) *effective problem identification and resolution lead to increased organizational effectiveness.*

Health care organizations do not live in a vacuum. Because of this fact, it is important to capture some of the future trends as they apply not only to health care but also to other organizations and society in general. An excellent resource is "Into the Twenty-first Century," a report from the World Future Society (1988). Some of the key points from this report include:

How Internal Consulting Can Increase Effectiveness 15

1. The most important area affecting America's future is education. Education will be the limiter of future technologies, human resource supplies, and the like.
2. With the aging of the population, definitions of the process of aging are needed. For example, the mandatory retirement age needs to be considered.
3. The bottom-line orientation that has been prevalent needs to give way to a longer-term view of the nation's future.

The report then continues to discuss seventy-one trends that it sees as important in the next twenty years. Specific trends impacting health care are that (1) significant developments in genetic engineering will take place; (2) transplant technology will become very sophisticated, and the ethical implications will become complex; and (3) there will be new computer diagnostic tools for physicians that will all but eliminate exploratory surgery. And, these trends are impacted by what will be and is happening in education, the aging population, changing societal values, and so on.

We believe firmly that the health care professional must be constantly aware of trends. Consequently, we have actively been involved in research looking at trends. Some key health care trends based on research we have done with health care professionals are:

Technological change. A constant theme in literature concerning the future is that of technological change. The costs of technology both provide for new treatment and diagnostic capabilities and drive up the cost of health care.

Continued emphasis on cost containment. There will probably be continued emphasis on cost containment efforts, although there will also be equal emphasis on generation of new revenue.

Aging populations, which will impact the work of health care. Populations' aging has two aspects. First, the patient population will get older, meaning that demands on the health care system will be greater. Second, health care professionals taking care of the population will get older.

Increasing acuity of health care patients. The future health care scene will involve sicker patients who require longer periods of stay.

Resurgence of self-care with the addition of high-tech devices. Patients of the future will be even better informed about their conditions than are patients today. Their access to data bases of information will increase. At the same time, use of home diagnostic tools will increase.

Continued shortages of health care professionals. The shortages will be in not only the nursing profession but also health care professions in general. This may drive health care organizations to be more driven by the human resources side of the business. In addition to long-range financial planning, long-range human resource planning will increase.

This factor is extremely important when considering the internal consultant role. A study conducted by SnowAntle, Stone, Vincelette, and Michaels (1989, pp. 146–148) reported that personnel turnover represents considerable costs in the continual recruitment and training of new employees and that the importance of doing well on the job is a key factor linked to increased organization tenure. This suggests the importance of providing employees with education, training, and opportunities (that is, successful internal consulting skills) necessary to maximize success experiences on the job, which overall lead to increased organization effectiveness.

Government regulation. Government regulation will continue to grow in the years ahead. This will probably include a major revision of the health care system. This also relates to the next trend.

Continuing changes in reimbursement. What form these changes will take is still unknown, but their reality is not. With increasing numbers of health care users being uninsured or underinsured and health care costs for businesses increasing rapidly, there is little doubt that there will be changes in the reimbursement system.

The above are some of the trends that we have found important. They are all aspects of one major trend about which we continually hear—the ability to manage change. If there is one trend to which almost all health care professionals agree, it is that change is ongoing. This means that we need to increase our ability to manage change and manage stress.

Internal Versus External Consultants

So far we have discussed the internal consultant almost completely. How does the internal consultant differ from the external consult? How are they similar or different? When do we decide to use the external consultant?

The answer to the first question is that the internal consultant functions within the organization, and the external consultant functions outside the organization. Both internal and external consultants have pluses and minuses, which this section will explore. First the internal consultant.

The strengths of internal consultant are:

1. *The internal consultant is a member of the organization and, as such, is very knowledgeable about the organization.* This is a major strength. We have all heard the statement "That's fine, but it would not work in our organization." Behind the statement is an important key—organizations do differ, and what works in one organization may not work in another. The internal consultant knows his or her organization and what will work or not work. He or she is an insider, a member of the family.

2. *Part of the internal consultant's knowledge has to do with how to get things done within the organization.* She or he knows to whom to talk and in what sequence. She or he knows that if a particular director is left out of the process, later that director will block the effort. In other words, the internal consultant understands the organizational politics and how to get things done.

Early on in my internal consulting experience, I learned this lesson the hard way. I had designed an intensive management development assessment process. As I proceeded to set up interviews with various vice-presidents, I discovered an interesting thing. None of them was available for the next six months. Their time was totally blocked out.

Then, about the time I was going to trash the project, I received a call from one vice-president asking me to come down for coffee. In the middle of the polite discussion over coffee, he gently let me know that I had "blown it." I had left a key player out of the process, and, if I wanted the process back on track, I needed to include that individual. I took his advice, and from that time on, my interviews came off without a hitch. More importantly, I learned an important internal consultant lesson—know who the key internal actors are and who needs to sanction the project.

3. *The internal consultant is not in the health care organization for a short-term consultation.* The internal consultant is not in the organization for a few days and then gone. He or she lives in the organization and has a long-term investment in the success of the program, since he or she will be there long after this one event. Perhaps even more important, the internal consultant is committed to the organization. Where the external consultant's primary allegiance is elsewhere, the internal consultant's primary allegiance is to the organization.

4. *The internal consultant has a history in the organization.* This is both positive and negative. Positively, the members of the organization know the internal consultant. If she or he has a record of getting things done and being a support to the department in getting things done, he or she will be well received.

The key for the internal consultant is to know and be part of the organization. The minuses of this are:

1. *The internal consultant may be too locked into the organization to fully understand or appreciate it.* The internal consultant may be blinded to the obvious problems because she or he is too close to the organization. The organizational norms have become invisible, like water to a fish or air to a bird—they are taken for granted.

2. *The internal consultant may get locked into some political battles and not be aware of these battles.* For example, two administrators may be warring and may try to use the internal consultant to gather information that will be damaging to the other party. The internal consultant can get caught in the cross fire and be rendered ineffective.

The internal consultant can also be seen as taking a side in the political battle. For example, a colleague of ours became embroiled in a political battle with nursing. As a result, she was

How Internal Consulting Can Increase Effectiveness   19

totally ineffective from that point on in working with the key nursing management. In fact, nursing stopped asking her for consults.

3. *The history the internal consultant brings may have negative impacts.* The internal consultant is an actor in the organization, meaning that he or she carries a significant history. If the department perceives the internal consultant as being ineffective and having really "messed up" with other departments, that perception will haunt the consultant.

4. *The internal consultant frequently takes for granted the "contracting" time with the internal client.* It is assumed that the internal consultant will accept each job and that turning down a job is not an option — the job is his or her responsibility. That means the internal consultant may not take the time necessary to really understand the client's needs and to fully identify the responsibilities and roles of the internal consultant and the client. Contracting can be sloppy because the internal consultant is "one of us."

The external consultant, in contrast, has the following strengths.

1. *The external consultant brings into the organization a fresh view of the organization.* An external consultant is not locked into the dynamics of the organization. She or he is like the small child in the story about the emperor's new clothes, in which, while all the adults are commenting on the fine new clothing the emperor has on, the child simply states, "But the emperor has no clothes on." The trance is broken, and all present see the reality. Similarly, the external consultant has a fresh view.

2. *The external consultant may bring experiences from a number of other organizations.* That means that the external consultant may have more options available.

3. *The external consultant will probably take more time to be sure that the contracting phase is done appropriately.* After all, his or her livelihood depends on it. The external consultant will be more specific about what he or she is willing to do and about time frames and associated costs.

4. *Since the external consultant is not associated with the organization for a long term, the organization may use the consultant to*

perform tasks that would be too politically sensitive for an internal consultant. For example, the external consultant might be used to study staffing and then make recommendations for staff enhancement or reduction. The external consultant can also be used to make discreet inquiries outside the organization. For example, a health care organization implementing a new computer system may use the external consultant to make vender inquiries that would otherwise alert the venders and result in a sales pitch.

What about minuses for the external consultant? The standard ones include:

1. *Since external consultants are not part of the organization, they can inadvertently make changes that have significant negative organizational impacts.* They can waste the organization's time by not knowing the organization.

2. *The external consultants' work can be rejected by the organization,* even though that work may be good. External consultants are not part of the organization, and sometimes as soon as their contract is ended, so is their work. Who among us has not waited for the consultant to leave our organization so we could get things done right!

3. *Because external consultants are not part of the organization, they may be self-serving in ways that are inappropriate.* A classical example is the consultant who creates ongoing work. Instead of assisting the organization in skilling itself, such a consultant creates even more dependencies within the organization.

Another example of this problem is the consultant who sells what he does best to the organization. In such a case, regardless of what the problems might be, the consultant's solution is always the same.

The above represent some of the differences between the external and the internal consultant. The important point is that the internal consultant is a family member, whereas the external consultant is not. Being part of the family brings all the "baggage" that being a member of that family means. In one family, that enhances the work of the individual; in another, that detracts from the work of the individual.

There is a place for the external consultant. Schein (1985,

p. 113) suggests that when making internal organizational assessments, one of the best "teams" is a combination of internal and external consultants. In such a team, the internal consultant and external consultant can build on their strengths and minimize their weaknesses. Because of the combined efforts, two predominant biases are avoided. The first is that of understanding the organization. The outsider enters with a basic ignorance of the organization. Without an insider to help interpret the organization and its needs, the outsider will miss important dynamics. The second is to overcome internal invisibility. The insider is blinded by the obvious. The insider is part of the system and has difficulty seeing it. The outsider can point to parts of the culture and ask, "Why do you do it that way?"

Our view is consistent with Schein's. We believe that the internal consultant role in combination with an external consultant role can result in a very effective working relationship. One example we have been working with recently is the design of a retreat for the board of directors of an organization. An outside consultant was hired to bring to the organization an outsider's experience and point of view. However, the design of the retreat was a joint effort between the outsider and the insider. The result—an effective use of the external and the internal consultant.

Change: Sidekick of the Internal Consultant

No book on internal consultants would be complete without discussing the impact of change. Why? Because much of what an internal consultant does relates to managing a change in the life of a department or the organization, whether that change is implementing a new policy or a new computer system. The result is that the internal consultant needs to have an understanding of the change process.

The change model of Kurt Lewin (1935, pp. 80ff.) is still the classical one. Lewin proposes three stages in the process of change. The first stage is *unfreezing the current conditions*. This means that the existing given conditions become open to question. It may involve something as simple as a policy that does not seem to do what needs to be done or as complex as a major organizational restructuring.

Typically, the unfreezing is focused in a problem. We have to make a change because if we do not we will have a serious problem or a problem that we currently have will become worse.

An accompanying point needs to be made here. We are all victims of habit. We become used to doing things in certain ways and will continue to do them that way until we are confronted with a need to change. Human behavior is like the law of physics that states that once a ball begins to move in a certain direction, it will continue in that direction until some other force contradicts it.

What does this mean? Change will be met with resistance. Even when serious problems are being encountered, suggestions for change will not be excluded from this resistance. Think for a moment about some couples that you know. Some couples live in a very unproductive, unaffirming relationship, and yet when an attempt is made to change the relationship, that attempt is highly resisted.

Again, the first stage in the change process is unfreezing the current conditions. What unfreezes? Something either within the organization or outside the organization. For example, a major unfreezing for health care organizations was the shift to prospective pricing systems. That external change in reimbursement has created a tremendous change within health care. Another example of an internal unfreezing is the hiring of a new CEO.

The second stage is *introducing the new change*. At an individual level, this means introducing the desired behavior. At an organization level, it means instituting the new changes. New strategies or technologies are introduced.

Again, expect that there will be resistance to change even if the change is generally desired. As an example, consider our experiences in introducing a new computer system. This was a major change in the life of the organization, and it was highly desired. Yet, as we moved into the process, we encountered significant resistance to the change, because it meant doing something differently.

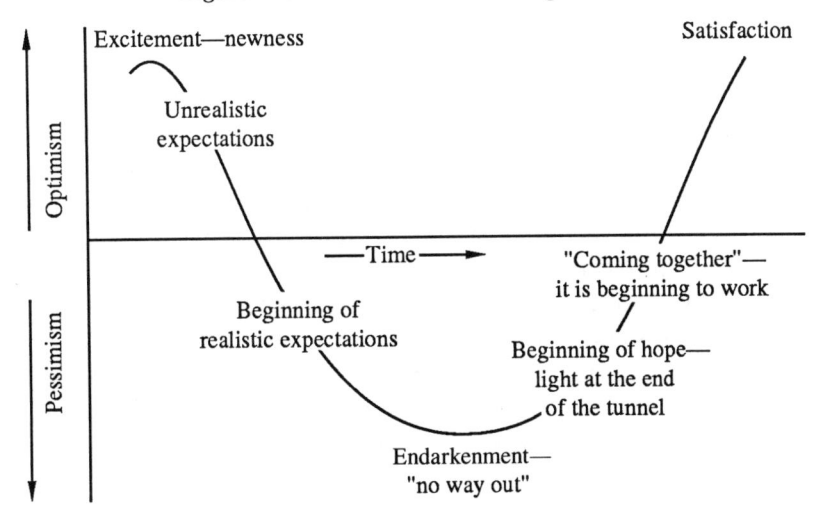

How Internal Consulting Can Increase Effectiveness 25

Figure 4. Revised Emotional Change Model.

1. Excitement
2. Beginning doubt
3. Total endarkenment
4. Glimpse of light
5. Optimism
6. Return to routine

We like to illustrate the emotional change cycle as shown in Figure 4. The revised model graphically illustrates the process as we see it happen. There is usually a literal sinking from optimism into pessimism. At some later point there is a turnaround when the "light at the end of the tunnel" is seen.

The revised emotional change model is dynamic. The model is changeable. There may be periods when the start point is pessimism. There may be periods of upward turning, when suddenly everything seems to be going downhill. The model provides a road map of a process, but we live that process through in many different ways.

Conclusion

This chapter has been about internal consulting. We have discussed what internal consulting is, its strengths and weaknesses, and the role of change. The role of the internal consultant is vital in today's health care world because of the human resource demands of health care organizations. Not only are health care organizations labor intensive; they also require that the human resources work closely together to produce a quality patient care product. The internal consultant both is impacted by and impacts change. The life of the internal consultant revolves around the management of change in either individual settings or across the organization.

Our basic message is this: internal consulting skills are vital to today's health care organizations. They are a key part of individuals' working together to provide quality patient care. Increasing the effectiveness of internal consulting means increasing the organizations' effectiveness.

2

The Roles and Skills of Internal Consultants

When you think of a consultant, what roles come to mind? Do you think of a person who is providing expert advice? Do you think of a person who knows more about an issue than the person with whom he or she is talking? Or do you think about a person who is more than fifty miles from home?

The purpose of this chapter is to explore consultant roles within the health care setting. When you complete this chapter, you will have a good sense of just how diverse the internal consultant role is.

This chapter has an important bias—that above all, *the consulting relationship is fundamentally that of helper and helpee*. The consultant has one purpose—*to assist the client* in the resolution of a problem, the prevention of a future problem, or the making of a decision. The consultant is seen as having a set of skills that are important for the client. These may be skills in assisting the client in thinking through the problem and arriving at a possible solution, that is, process consultation skills or skills in actually addressing the problem or providing technical skills for the client. The key is that the client is someone who is seeking help, and the consultant is someone who is offering help to the client.

Reducing the consultant role to one basic role, that of helper, means that the starting place for understanding the consultant role is understanding the helper-helpee relationship.

This chapter begins by discussing this relationship, and later chapters will expand on this theme.

In this chapter we will first discuss the helper-helpee relationship as core to the work of internal consulting. Internal consulting is simply effective helping. Second, we will translate that helping relationship into common roles for the internal consultant. Sometimes when you need a helper, you need someone to tell you what to do. At other times, someone's telling you what to do is the worst possible treatment. Sometimes you need someone who will listen to you and help you think through the problem and arrive at an answer. Internal consultant roles can be seen as being on a continuum from telling you what needs to happen to thinking through the problem with you.

Third, we present a model for understanding what consultant role fits best with what helper need. This is an important point. We believe that the key to successful internal consulting is being able to shift the internal consultant role according to the particular client problem and needs. Again, that means that sometimes the internal consultant needs to be directive and at other times must be a listener. The model that we present is a decision tree for use when trying to decide what role will be most effective.

The Helper-Helpee Role

Take a few minutes before you read further in this chapter and think about the following questions:

Remember the last time you needed to ask someone for help or assistance. What was that experience like for you? What feelings did you have? Was it easy or hard for you to do?

Now think back to the last time that someone came to you for help. What was that experience like for you? What were the feelings that went along with it? Was it easy or difficult for you to do?

The core of the internal consultant role is helping. Whether the internal consultant is offering technical advice or emotional support, help is being offered. The client has sought out the internal consultant for some reason. Basically, that

The Roles and Skills of Internal Consultants 29

means the client feels that there is some type of deficient; something is not right! It might be an immediate problem. It might be an expected problem. It might be simply a gap between what is and some more desired state. Whatever the reason, the relationship is that of helper and helpee.

Think back to the questions at the beginning of this section. They represent two sets of responses. The first concerns what it feels like to ask for help. In competitive health care organizations, asking for help may be a very difficult thing to do that could be seen as a weakness. If the asking individual has difficulty asking for help, the chances the request will be made become more remote. Some individuals believe that to ask for help is a sign of incompetence. Reflect on your responses. In your belief system, is it acceptable to ask for help from others? Or do you think less of yourself when you ask for help? The internal consultant needs to know what his or her own comfort level is in asking for help. If the internal consultant is not comfortable in asking for help, he or she may unknowingly communicate that to the client. The result can be a confused and unproductive consult.

The second set of questions focuses on how you respond when you are asked for help. For many in the helping professions, this is a very comfortable position. Being asked for help is very ego gratifying—it implies that someone sees us as useful and competent. We are needed instead of needing. The internal consultant needs to be aware of her or his need to be needed. This need can get in the way of the client's resolving problems.

Review your responses to the questions at the beginning of this section and think for a moment about the implications of your responses for the internal consultant role. In Chapter Ten we will discuss in greater depth some of the issues of the helper-helpee relationship.

Types of Problems

We differentiate three levels of problems that are brought to the internal consultant. We refer to them as first-, second-, and third-degree problems.

A first-degree problem occurs when the client is seeking a better way of doing something. For example, human resources might be exploring the benefit package and considering more attractive benefits, or nursing might be trying to identify new recruitment strategies. The search is for something better. There is no real need to change the present conditions.

A second-degree problem is one that has become an irritant and needs to be addressed. Perhaps the issue is increasing turnover for the past few months. Perhaps it is an unexpected census drop-off that needs to be explored. Unlike a first-degree problem, a second-degree problem requires attention. The oil light on your car is an analogy. Its blinking on and off may or may not indicate a serious problem, but it certainly warrants your attention.

A third-degree problem is one where survival is at stake. The issue cannot be ignored without the survival of the department, function, or organization being called into question. The problem demands attention. It is like the oil light that stays on in the car when the engine is beginning to smoke. Action must be taken.

Within the health care organization, a third-degree problem might be infection rates that suddenly begin to inexplicably increase. It might be a financial indicator that has reached a crisis level. The important point is that a crisis has been reached that needs the full attention of the department or organization.

The internal consultant working with a client needs to be aware of the degree of problem being discussed. Different degrees of problems will require that the internal consultant play different roles. A problem that is simply the search for a better idea will not require the same rigor and immediate attention as will a crisis.

We will discuss this more later in this chapter as we explore when to use different roles. For now, take a few moments and consider the following questions.

Think about your recent work experience. What is an example of each type of problem (first degree, second degree, and third degree) and how did you change your response to the problem?

The Roles and Skills of Internal Consultants 31

The Starting Point: Perceptions

The core of any helping relationship is perceptions. Perceptions are what trigger our attitudes and behaviors toward another person or situation. Our belief is that it is critical for the helper to understand his or her perceptions of what it means to be in a helping relationship.

The real work of the internal consultant is understanding the world of the client. Without that understanding, the internal consultant will never be able to effectively address the client's problems. However, the paradox is that in order to understand the other person's world, the consultant must first understand her or his own world of perceptions.

Imagine an internal consultant with no self-understanding. Such a person is very likely to project his or her needs on the other person in ways that will eventually interfere with effective helping. For example, if I have a need to be needed by the client, probably that need will eventually get in the way of my being an effective helper. If we think of a lack of self-understanding as a filter system that blocks out certain signals from the client, then the tighter our filter, the less we will be able to see the problem clearly from the client's point of view.

Our belief is that the greatest tool that the internal consultant brings to the setting is his or her own self-understanding and -awareness. That self-understanding will allow for clear contracting and decision making within the consulting relationship and will allow the internal consultant to make most effective use of his or her technical skills.

One model that we have found very useful in understanding perceptions and how they are formed is that of percept language (Weir and Weir, 1985). Figure 5 illustrates our rendition of the percept language model.

Percept language begins with filter 1 — our sensory channels. Think about it for a moment. The journey to forming a perception and a response to an event or a person begins with sensations channeled to our brain via our sensory inputs. The sensory inputs include such things as sight, hearing, smell, touch, and so on. If our physical hearing is not accurate, we may

Figure 5. Percept Language Model.

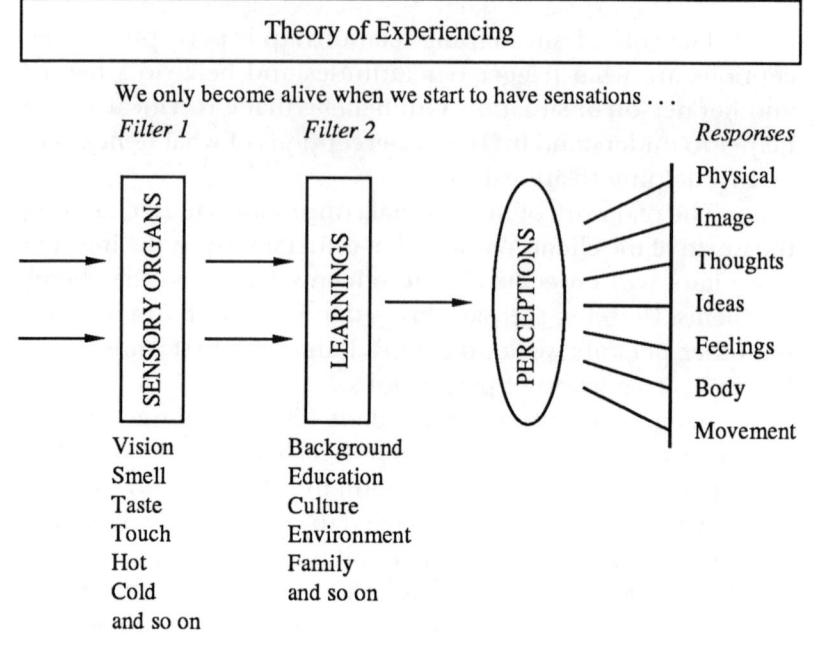

Theory of Experiencing

We only become alive when we start to have sensations . . .

Filter 1 — SENSORY ORGANS → *Filter 2* — LEARNINGS → PERCEPTIONS → *Responses*: Physical, Image, Thoughts, Ideas, Feelings, Body Movement

Filter 1:
Vision
Smell
Taste
Touch
Hot
Cold
and so on

Filter 2:
Background
Education
Culture
Environment
Family
and so on

Source: Weir and Weir, 1985. Used with permission.

miss important data and form an incorrect response to the client. If our seeing is limited, we may miss physically seeing a particular item. Filter 1 is our physical limitations to receiving the sensations from which we form perceptions.

Filter 2 is our past learnings that impact the passage of sensations. We may have learned to not hear certain things—for example, if something "not nice" is said about someone, we may not hear it. We may have learned to not see certain things—for example, if two people are in conflict, we may have learned not to see the conflict. The important point is that each of us has formed certain assumptions about ourselves and the world around us that influence what sensations we will allow to pass through the filter to form our perceptions. The learnings that we have picked up from our environment form this second filter.

After data pass through the two filters, the individual

The Roles and Skills of Internal Consultants

forms a perception. From that perception, action will follow. The action may be a thought, physical movement, feeling, or something else. The behavior we see in ourselves and in our clients is a result of this process. Behaviors are based on perceptions, and perceptions are limited and formulated by what the two filters have allowed through.

Of special importance for the internal consultant are her or his learnings about what it means to be in a helping relationship. What does it mean to be a helper? Can a helper help someone and let that person develop? For example, if the internal consultant has a need to be a helper, she or he may need to keep the client in a dependency role. Or, if the internal consultant sees asking for help as a weakness, he or she will look down on the client for needing help. Our past learnings greatly impact the helping relationship, and they impact how effective the internal consultant will be in assisting the client.

Understanding perceptions as the basis for behavior has two important implications for the internal consultant. The first implication is self-understanding. The greater the internal consultant's self-awareness, the greater the probability he or she will be effective. Our earlier comments regarding the importance of self-knowledge and self-awareness emphasize this point. Lack of self-knowledge can be an internal consultant's blind spot. Blind spots are the areas where the internal consultant will find difficulty.

One useful tool in increasing self-awareness is that of the Johari window (Luft and Ingham, 1973, pp. 114–119) (see Figure 6). The Johari window is a tool for increasing self-awareness and discovery of blind spots in self-perception.

The Johari window has four parts. The first part contains things I know about myself that others know about me. This is the "public" me, the part of me known to the people at work and to myself. I like people, and they know that I like people. We have common information.

The second part contains things I know about myself that others do not know. This is the hidden part of me. I know this aspect of myself, but others do not know it. Perhaps it is as simple as a hobby of which others do not know. Maybe it is not

Figure 6. Johari Window Model.

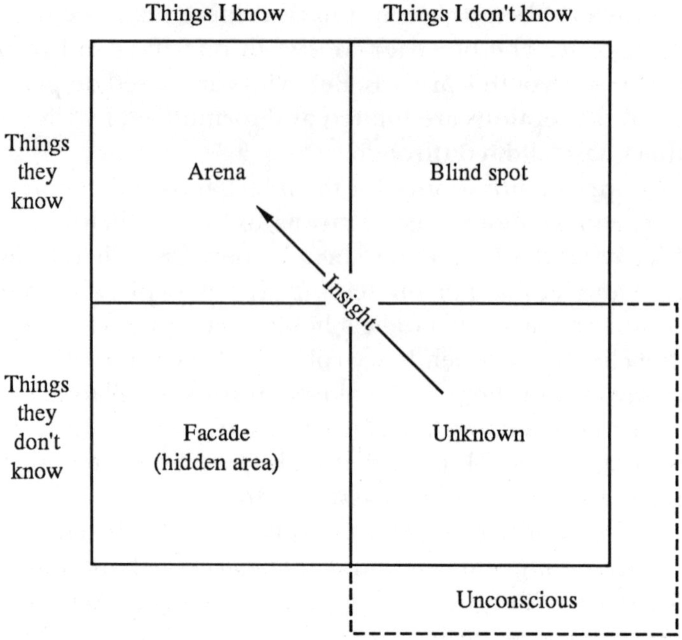

	Things I know	Things I don't know
Things they know	Arena	Blind spot
Things they don't know	Facade (hidden area)	Unknown

Insight (arrow from center toward Arena)

Unconscious (dashed area extending beyond)

Source: Jones and Pfeiffer, 1973. Used with permission.

letting others know about some family secret. This is the part of me that I keep secret.

The third part contains things others know about me that I do not know. This is the part of me that is hidden from myself but obvious to others. There will always be some aspects of myself that others will see that I may not. This area is especially important for the internal consultant. It is very important to develop feedback loops to minimize this area. There is nothing worse than having things happen behind you of which you are unaware. These are the blind spots.

The fourth part contains things I do not know about me that others do not know about me. These are my unknown areas. A psychologist might call this the unconscious. Neither I nor others are aware of these things.

Take a moment and think about the following items.

The Roles and Skills of Internal Consultants

1. Identify three things about yourself that you know and that you know others know.
2. Identify three things about yourself that you know but that are not common knowledge to others.
3. What is something about you that you think others know that you are not sure about? (This gets tricky. If you have trouble with this question, talk to a friend or two. Ask them what they know about you that they think you do not know.)
4. What is something about yourself that you learned in the past two weeks that you never realized before that you think others also did not know.

One of the tasks of the internal consultant is to continually be exploring ways to increase awareness of blind spots and the unconscious. These blind spots will always be there—that is part of the human mystery—and yet, the task for the internal consultant is to be constantly learning.

The second implication has to do with the internal consultant's understanding of the client. The client's behavior and attitude are understandable when time is taken to understand the perceptions behind the attitude or behavior. Consider, for example, an internal consultant working with a client who becomes quite outraged at something. Instead of simply discounting the client or his outrage, the internal consultant should try to get inside the client's world and understand what the outrage is about. When we take the time to think the issue through from the client's point of view, we normally arrive at a new understanding of the situation.

The foundation of the internal consultant role in a health care organization is that of a helping relationship. The next section will build on this foundation by identifying specific behaviors that are part of a number of helping roles.

Multiple Roles

Once again, think back to the number of times you have been in a helper or a helpee role. You will recognize that what worked in that relationship varied from time to time. In one setting the helper was directive. In another setting the helper was more supportive. The lesson—there are many different helping roles for the internal consultant.

A number of descriptions of consultant roles also can be seen as internal consultant roles. Perhaps the classic is from Margulies and Raia (1978, p. 113). Margulies and Raia discuss the consultant role from the perspective of task orientation or process orientation.

We will take a few minutes to discuss the model and its implication for the internal consultant. We will discuss the two approaches with regard to several variables, beginning with the characteristics of the task orientation. If you approach a client using the task orientation, the following will be some characteristics of your work:

1. *Problem verification.* The consultant collects the data and then presents them to the client.
2. *Problem solving.* The consultant is in charge. The consultant designs the research and develops the solutions for the client.
3. *Feedback.* The consultant feeds back the data to the client and provides expert data interpretation.
4. *Utilization of research.* The data collected become the foundation for specific recommendations.
5. *Involvement.* The involvement of the consultant is primarily with the problem to be solved.
6. *Relationship to client.* The relationship between consultant and client is minimal. It is usually detached and distant, businesslike and distant.
7. *Systems approach.* The consultant is concerned with the implications of the problem for other parts of the organization.

The process facilitator has a different set of characteristics. If you approach a client using this orientation, you will do and look for things in somewhat different ways. These include:

The Roles and Skills of Internal Consultants

1. *Problem verification.* The problem is verified by various means. The client's feelings and thoughts regarding the problem are considered valid data.
2. *Problem solving.* The interest of the process facilitator is in enhancing the problem-solving capabilities of the system within which he or she is working.
3. *Feedback.* The process facilitator provides multiple sources of data and assists the client in arriving at conclusions. The client is very much part of the interpretation of the data.
4. *Utilization of research.* The goal is to get the client to use and apply the learnings from the data.
5. *Involvement.* The involvement has to do with the problem but also with the people and the system.
6. *Relationship to client.* The process facilitator is involved with the client. The connection is typically a long one.
7. *Systems approach.* The process consultant is concerned with relationships among many departments within the organization and works at clearing channels of communication between those departments.

The internal consultant who functions from the task orientation will have specific behaviors. The following scenario is an illustration.

> The administrator contacted us and requested that we analyze turnover within the fiscal departments because he sensed that turnover was unreasonably high in these departments.
>
> We accepted the task and laid out a very task-oriented plan. Our first step was to conduct an hour-long program for the fiscal managers to review the causes and consequences of turnover, present predictor variables associated with turnover, and discuss industry turnover statistics.
>
> Our second step was to go to the departments and explore the problem of turnover as it appeared in the individual departments. Again, we told the managers what we wanted and when we wanted it. Exit interviews were

reviewed, and focus groups were held with those within the department who had stayed and with some of the leavers. Next, we did a multivariate analysis for the information and came up with predictor variables for turnover within the departments.

Our last step was to prepare a detailed report for the administrator including recommendations for actions and next steps.

You can see from this example how the consultant functions as a technical expert.

An internal consultant functioning from a process orientation will behave much differently than one using a task orientation. The following scenario illustrates a process orientation.

The nursing director asked for assistance in working through the decision whether to hire new graduate nurses to fill several vacant positions in the nursing areas. The project stretched over several months and had many joint meetings with the nursing administrator and several nursing directors. Our first suggestion was to involve the human resource department in the discussion as they would be a key department in the recruitment decision. In this situation we gathered information from other community resources regarding their graduate nurse programs, and we worked with several universities.

The key is that as we worked with the nursing directors, we provided thoughts and ideas on how to go about the task, but our primary focus was on the process rather than on being directive. In the end, we provided the nursing directors with a process for arriving at a decision rather than with a given answer. The client was walked through a process rather than being given a solution.

The Margulies and Raia model (see Figure 7) illustrates a range of consultant roles along the continuum from technical expert (task orientation) to process facilitator. We developed our model based on our experience with the Margulies and Raia

The Roles and Skills of Internal Consultants

Figure 7. Range of Consultative Roles.

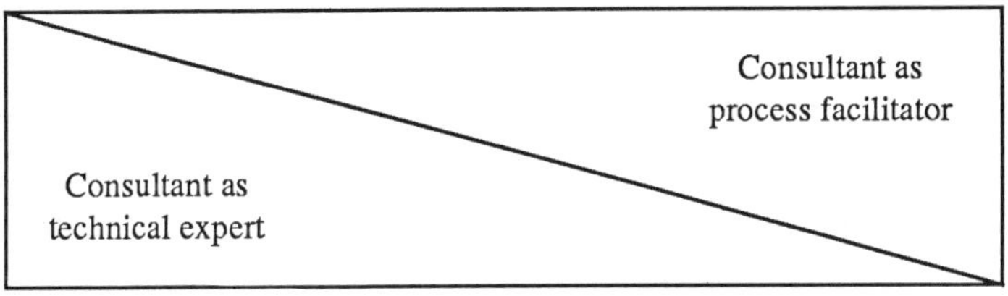

[Diagram: A rectangle divided diagonally, with "Consultant as technical expert" labeled on the lower-left and "Consultant as process facilitator" labeled on the upper-right.]

Source: Margulies and Raia, 1978. Used with permission.

model and on the Consultation Skills Inventory (1976) and McLagan (1983).

The internal consultant can function in many roles ranging from the expert at one end of the continuum to the process facilitator at the other end, and there are a multitude of combinations in between. At one phase of the consulting cycle, the internal consultant may be more of a technical expert. At another point, he or she may be more process oriented.

Take a moment and think about the following questions. As you read over the two listings of characteristics by Margulies and Raia, with which listing do you most closely identify? What is an example of how this has been lived out in your work? How has this been useful for you, and how has it not been useful?

Lippitt and Lippitt (1986, pp. 57ff.) provide a different continuum for consulting roles. Their continuum is from nondirective to directive. The question asked is: To what degree is the client being directive, and to what degree is the internal consultant directed? When the internal consultant is most directive she or he is an advocate for the client. When the internal consultant is least directive, she or he is a process consultant for the client.

Using this model, the multiple roles for the internal consultant become (from directive to nondirective):

1. *Advocate.* In this role, the consultant is actively engaged with the client in directing in the problem-solving process and in proposing guidelines to be considered. An example of this is the information resource internal consultant who has discovered that the client is not using the information system correctly. The internal consultant as advocate in this setting becomes very directive about what the problem is and how to resolve it.

2. *Information specialist.* In this role, the client defines the problem and the objectives of the consultation. The consultant then proceeds to provide the client with options.

For example, in designing a computer program for a client, as the internal consultant I simply solve the client's problem. The client tells me the desired end results, and I do the work. I then present the client with the solution.

One problem with this role was mentioned earlier. In most cases the presenting problem is not the real problem. If the internal consultant moves too quickly, the result can be time wasted because of working on the wrong problems.

A second problem with this role is the well-known game of "yes...but." The internal consultant is in the position of suggesting solutions and finds that the client is simply saying, "Yes... but that will not work." For those of you who have not experienced the "yes...but" game, it goes something like this:

Consultant: What I think you should do is bring in a management engineer to review your work flow. That will help you determine where the problems are.

Client: Yes, but I do not have a budget that will allow for an external consultant.

Consultant: There are a couple of other managers who might be able to assist you with this. How about talking with them on how they worked with this problem in their area?

Client: Well, that sounds good, but I do not think they have done much better than I have. In fact, they talked to me about it.

Consultant: How about having me continue to work with you and design the process?

Client: Yes... but, I know you are busy and...

You know that you are caught up with "yes...but" when you are working harder at the solutions than the client is, and every idea that comes up is rejected. You find yourself leaving the client feeling frustrated and confused.

3. *Trainer and educator.* In this role, the consultant designs

training experience of some type that addresses the need of the client group. Perhaps it is a training session on a new feature of the telephone system. The internal consultant presents the program to the client group as part of the change process from the old to the new.

4. *Joint problem solver.* Another role is that of joint problem solver. The client and the consultant collaborate to determine what the problem is and how best to direct its resolution.

A good example is that of team building within a department. The internal consultant and the department work together to come up with the key problems and possible solutions. The effort is collaborative.

5. *Identifier of alternatives and linker to resources.* Many times the consultant's role is to simply help the client link with someone else who can provide help. For example, a personal computer consultant may link two individuals within the organization who use the same word-processing program. The client having trouble with the word-processing program is matched with someone who is using the package and may have a solution.

Such networking is a key feature of the internal consultant. Many of the audiences for this book were selected because they have access to wide segments of the organization. They are able and welcome to appear in other departments. For example, the chaplain has access to most parts of the organization. This means he or she knows much about what is going on. A very important function of the internal consultant is linking together those who have particular problems with those who have possible solutions.

6. *Fact finder.* The fact finder is the researcher. In this role, the consultant goes about finding information that the client needs. An example is a turnover study in which we are engaged. The client used us to research a problem and then provide him with data. The internal consultant role here is simple—find the data, organize them, and deliver them to the client.

7. *Process consultant.* When the internal consultant is in the process consultant role, the consultant and the client jointly work together to diagnose the problem. The way the client does his work is part of what is reviewed. Questions such as "How is the client behavior keeping the problem a problem?" will occur.

The focus is not always directly on the problem; it is also sometimes on how the client is going about trying to resolve the problem. The consultant's objective is to give the client the skills needed to correct the problem in the future.

Take a moment with the roles discussed by Lippitt and Lippitt. Think about your work as an internal consultant and about what percentage of your internal consultant time you spend in each role. In which of these roles do you spend the most time? What is the strength of that particular role? What is its down side?

The message from both Lippitt and Lippitt and Margulies and Raia is that there are multiple consultant roles to which the internal consultant must be sensitive.

The Four Roles

The discussion so far has shown the roles on a continuum either from task to process or from directive to nondirective. Our approach moves from using one dimension (a continuum) to using two dimensions. Our framework is built on the work of Hersey and Blanchard (1977) on situational leadership. The first dimension is the amount of directiveness the internal consultant demonstrates, similar to the Lippitt and Lippitt continuum. The second dimension is the amount of leadership, that is, subjective involvement with the client, that the internal consultant demonstrates. This is more on the process side of the equation, as discussed by Margulies and Raia. These two dimensions are seen in Figure 8.

The degree of directiveness is the degree to which the consultant initiates the relationship and provides the specifics with regard to who, what, when, where, how much, and desired outcomes. Is the internal consultant doing more talking than the client? Is the consultant saying what needs to be done, when it needs to be done, who needs to do it, and so on? Directive behavior means the consultant is taking the lead.

The degree of relationship has to do with the amount of relationship the consultant has with the client. Relationship refers to the consultant's investing himself or herself in the

The Roles and Skills of Internal Consultants

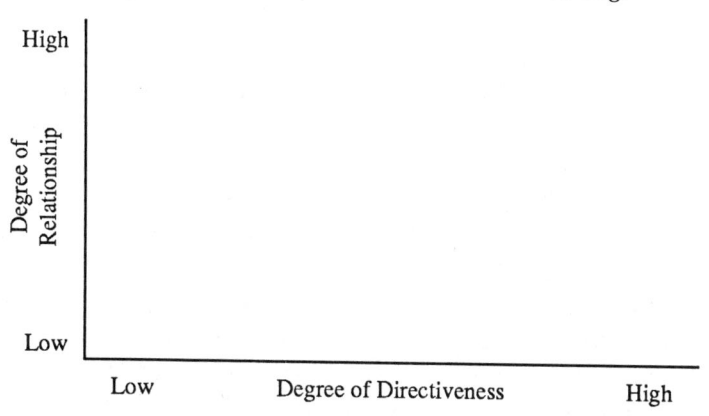

Figure 8. Two Dimensions of Internal Consulting.

client. The consultant is not interested only in the particular problem that has been identified. He or she is interested in the client and in the relationship of the client to the rest of the organization. A high degree of relationship means that the internal consultant is willing to be influenced by as well as to influence the client.

The result of this two-dimensional model would be an infinite number of consultant-client relationship roles. However, we would like to use four primary roles. These are shown in Figure 9.

Figure 9. Four Primary Internal Consulting Roles.

Facilitator	Counselor
Delegator	Director

The *director* is seen in the technical consultation where the internal consultant is very directive. Like a director of a stage production, the internal consultant is directing the activities: the client needs to do these five things by this time with these results and with the involvement of these people. It might be the hospital information system representative who has come in to resolve a particular departmental problem. The expert is there to direct. Communication is one-way, from the internal consultant to the client.

The *counselor* is a combination of expert and facilitator. The counselor will be directive in asking the client questions and inviting the client to share thoughts and suggestions as the consult continues. However, the counselor is still very much in charge of the questions and the process of what is happening. Communication is a bit more two-way, but the consultant decides what is and is not addressed.

The important aspect of this role is that the client is still being directed. However, more is invested in the relationship. The internal consultant is investing more by giving more information to the client and by providing the client with more opportunity to react to the process. However, the directiveness still comes from the internal consultant.

The *facilitator* moves into a collaborative relationship with the client. Together they explore the problem and arrive at potential solutions. In the process, the skills of the client group are enhanced. The internal consultant will leave the client "smarter" as a result of an effective facilitation. At times the client takes the lead and is directive, and at times the consultant. Communication is clearly two-way, and the client has ample opportunity to influence the consultant.

Perhaps the distinguishing feature of this role is that it is open to mutual influence. The client can influence the internal consultant, and the internal consultant can influence the client.

The *delegator* role is interesting. Although it may initially seem that there is no real need for the delegator role, there are settings where it may be very useful. As delegator, the consultant takes a definite nondirective role. It may be a matter of observ-

The Roles and Skills of Internal Consultants

ing client meetings and then providing an occasional suggestion. The relationship and the directiveness are minimal.

Take a moment to think about the strengths and minuses of each role (director, counselor, facilitator, and delegator).

Each of the styles has pluses and minuses, benefits and costs. A director is needed when immediate action and someone to provide immediate directions are needed. However, people around a director often do not learn to develop but instead wait for someone to come in and rescue them.

A counselor involves the client group to a greater extent and can be more palatable than a director. The counselor provides direction but also engages in a discussion with the client. However, the client can sometimes become confused as to when the counselor is asking for input and when the counselor is telling what needs to be done. It may be participative management with a hidden agenda.

The facilitator is strongest in helping the client think through the problem and the best way to address it. There is mutual give-and-take between the facilitator and the client. However, this means that the client may not get the expert advice that was sought.

A delegator allows the client much autonomy. There is no separation issue since the consultant lets the client grow the way the client wants to grow. Sometimes, however, the client may need more directiveness than he gets from a delegator.

We believe that these roles are all appropriate, depending on the setting. Our axiom is: all roles are useful, and not every role will be useful in all settings. Think about this for a moment. All the roles have a place. However, not every role will be as effective for a particular situation as for the next.

That leads to a question: Assuming that the consultant has the option of choosing from which role she or he will function, what criteria can be used to select the appropriate role? What decision process can be gone through to increase the probability of a good decision?

Lippitt and Lippitt (1986, pp. 71ff.) suggest the following

factors be considered when determining what roles the consultant needs to take:

1. The nature of the contract. What is the agreement about roles in the contract? As we discuss contracting in a later chapter, we will focus the importance of agreeing on who will be taking what role in the consultation.
2. Goals. What are the goals of the consulting relationship? It is important that the internal consultant's early work be focused on understanding the client's goals.
3. Norms and standards of the client system and the consultant.
4. Personal limitations and inclinations of the consultant.
5. What worked before.
6. Whether the work is external or internal.
7. Events: for example, leadership change in the organization.

The Lippitt and Lippitt criteria are useful in making a decision regarding what role the internal consultant should take. However, the question is left open ended. We would like to take it a step further.

Let us go back to the concept we discussed earlier—that roles are a choice. Given that the consultant is most interested in a successful helping relationship, the key is what role the client needs at that time. We are talking about the client's needs as driving the selection of the consulting role. For example, if the client is in a crisis, the appropriate internal consultant role may be the director, providing directive behavior. If the client is in an early phase of problem identification, the appropriate role may be the counselor. Our point is simple: the client's needs are the driving factor in selecting the most effective consultant role.

The decision tree in Figure 10 is adapted from a model by Jones and Bearley (1986). This model provides the consultant with a specific decision matrix for deciding what internal consultant role to use with a specific client at a specific time. The model has the following components:

1. *Time.* Time has to do with the urgency of the consultation. Is it one that needs to happen immediately, or can it be

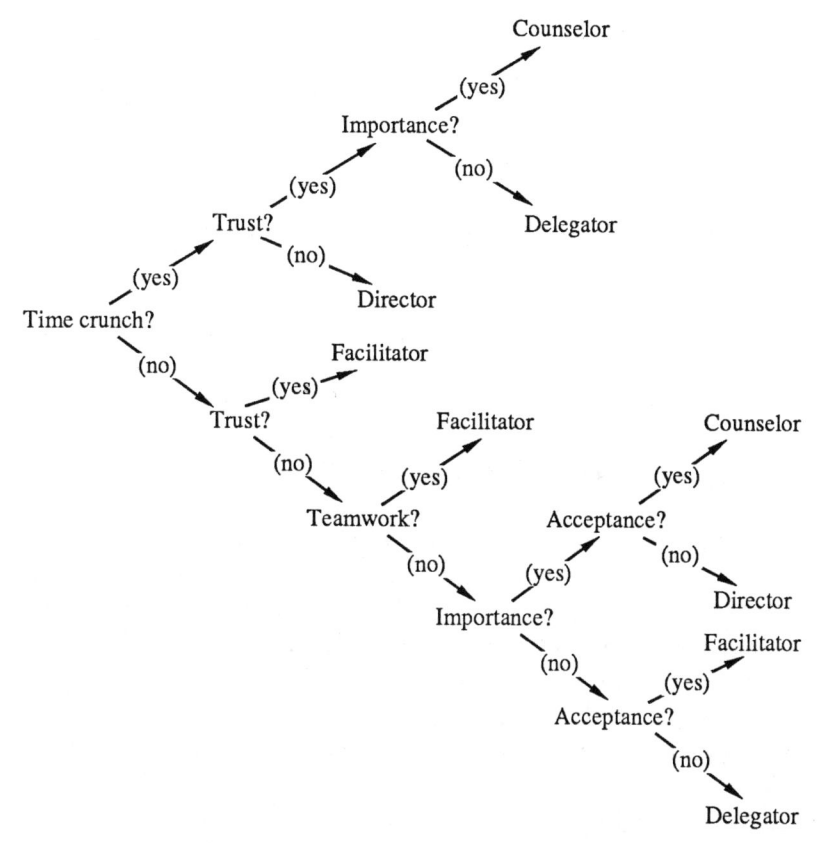

The Roles and Skills of Internal Consultants   47

Figure 10. Consulting Role Decision Tree.

```
                                              Counselor
                                            ↗
                                      (yes)
                              Importance?
                          ↗           ↘
                    (yes)              (no)
              Trust?                        ↘
           ↗        ↘                        Delegator
     (yes)          (no)
                       ↘
Time crunch?            Director
     ↘
     (no)               Facilitator
        ↘            ↗
         Trust? (yes)
              ↘                Facilitator              Counselor
              (no)           ↗                        ↗
                        (yes)                    (yes)
                 Teamwork?              Acceptance?
                       ↘           ↗          ↘
                       (no)   (yes)           (no)
                                                  ↘
                          Importance?              Director
                                ↘                  Facilitator
                                (no)             ↗
                                   ↘        (yes)
                                   Acceptance?
                                        ↘
                                        (no)
                                           ↘
                                           Delegator
```

Source: Adapted from Jones and Bearley, 1986.

done at leisure? Is there a time crunch involved? The more critical time is as a factor, the more important the directive role.

Refer back to our earlier discussion of types of problems. Typically, third-degree problems need to be responded to immediately, as they have associated time crunches.

2. *Trust.* Do the people involved in the consultation trust each other? Do they trust the internal consultant? This becomes a significant fact for the consultation. If trust is low, it limits the amount of role options available to the internal consultant.

3. *Teamwork.* To what degree does teamwork come into

the consultation? Is teamwork a desired outcome for the consultation? Does it matter?

A side question is: Does the consultant have as part of his or her agenda the intent to leave the client smarter than when he or she came into the organization? If so, team building may be an important agenda.

4. *Importance.* How important is the consultation to the organization? Does it provide clear benefits or harm to the organization? Again, the assumption is that consultations can be assessed on their importance for the organization.

5. *Acceptance.* How important is it for the client group to have high acceptance of the resolution? Will the client group have high levels of feelings about the decision or the process of the decision making?

Given these five criteria, the following decision choices can be made:

Director is an excellent role decision when:

(1) There is a time crunch and there are low levels of trust in the client group. In such a setting, the most appropriate role is one intervening as a director. John Wayne is needed to come to town and clean up the place!

(2) When there is no time crunch, trust is low, teamwork is not an issue, the decision is important, and acceptance is not a significant issue. Again, here we need a leader who will say who will do what when and what the results need to be.

Counselor is a useful style when:

(1) There is a time crunch, there are high levels of trust in the client system, and the decision is important. Because the group members trust one another, the counselor can let the group reach more joint decisions.

(2) There is no time crunch, trust is minimal, teamwork is not an agenda item, and the decision and its acceptance are important. The key in this is the importance and acceptance of the decision.

Facilitator is a useful role when:

(1) There is no time crunch, and there is significant trust in the client system. This means there is breathing time. There is

The Roles and Skills of Internal Consultants 49

time to think about the decision. We prefer to have consultations in this type of mode—there is no crisis driving us.

(2) There is no time crunch, there is minimal trust, and teamwork becomes an agenda. This is an excellent time to build the team. The time pressures are off, and there can be time to work together in ways that build trust.

(3) There is no time crunch, trust is minimal, teamwork is not an agenda, the importance is not high, and acceptance of the consultation is important. Here facilitation is important as a way of defusing blocks and talking issues through.

Delegator is most useful when:

(1) There is a time crunch, there is trust, but the importance is minimal. Let someone else do it! For most of us in health care, we need to be focused on important issues.

(2) There is no time crunch, trust is minimal, teamwork is not an agenda, importance is low, and acceptance is low. The only question we have is: Why are we spending time working on it?

The questionnaire in Exhibit 1 may be used to make a decision regarding the internal consultant role. You can use it to make decisions at various points in the consultation process.

Reflections on the Decision Tree

The decision tree represents one way to reach the decision on what internal consultant role to use. However, it needs to be seen as a starting point. As the client relationship develops, the roles will shift. For example, the ideal internal consultant–helpee relationship begins with dependency of the client on the consultant for some type of service. The client needs something the consultant has. As the relationship matures, that dependency should shift as well. When the client relationship is finished, the client should no longer be dependent on the consultant. The graph in Figure 11 depicts this shift in dependency.

The important point is that the decision tree can be used as a starting point for the consultation, but it also needs to be updated throughout the consultation. As the consultation ma-

50 Consultation Skills for Health Care Professionals

Exhibit 1. Internal Consultant Role Questionnaire.

The following questionnaire is a tool that may be used to make a decision regarding the internal consultant role. You can use it to make decisions at various points in the consultation process.

Take a few moments and focus an example of a specific consultation in your mind. Describe it below:

Respond to each of the following statements as you think about the consulting example. Circle the letter(s) that best describes your sense of where the consultant probably was on each dimension.

1. *Time.* The need for the immediate action in the consultation is
       High   Low
       T   t
2. *Trust.* The trust level between the consultant and the client is
       High   Low
       TR   tr
3. *Teamwork.* The desire for teamwork to be an important outcome of the consultation is
       High   Low
       TW   tw
4. *Importance.* The importance of the consultation for the organization is
       High   Low
       I   i
5. *Acceptance.* The importance of the client group's accepting the decision once it has been made is
       High   Low
       A   a

Scoring

Take your responses to the questions and put them in the blanks in front of the dimensions.

    ___ Time
    ___ Trust
    ___ Teamwork
    ___ Importance
    ___ Acceptance

Now match that set of responses with the following set:

Director	T,tr,tw,i,a
	t,tr,tw,I,a
Counselor	T,TR,tw,I,a
	t,tr,tw,I,A
Facilitator	t,TR,tw,i,a
	t,tr,TW,i,a
	t,tr,tw,i,A
Delegator	T,TR,tw,i,a
	t,tr,tw,i,a

Based on this analysis, the role most likely to occur is:

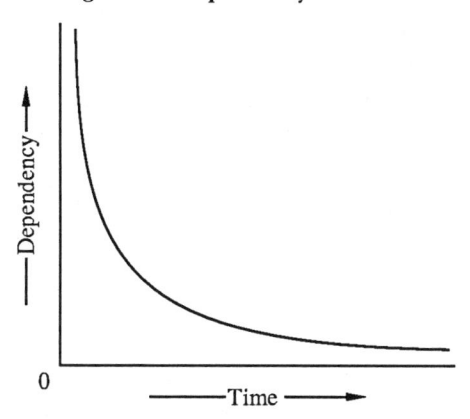

The Roles and Skills of Internal Consultants 51

Figure 11. Dependency Versus Time.

[Graph showing a decreasing curve with Dependency on the y-axis and Time on the x-axis, starting high and asymptotically approaching zero.]

tures, the roles will change. We will discuss this in greater detail in Part Two on the consultation process.

Chapter Three provides an overview of the consultation process. At each decision point presented in the consultation process, the internal consultant needs to ask: What role do I need to take for the next step of the process? Is my current role facilitating getting the necessary job done, or is it getting in the way?

Changes in the client system also may cause the consultant to shift roles. For example, a problem that was not a time crunch now becomes one of time shortage. The decision tree allows for changes in the internal consultant–client relationship based on the changing nature of the setting.

One last comment. We are aware that our model for the selection of consultant role is simple and has its limitations. However, it provides a way to think through the appropriate role. The internal consultant can use it when trying to determine the most effective role for the specific consultation into which he or she is going.

Summary

This chapter has identified several important beliefs that we have regarding consulting roles. First, the core of the internal consultant–client relationship is a helper-helpee role. It is vital that the internal consultant recognize this helper-helpee dynamic. Second, the internal consultant's self-awareness and self-understanding are vital to a successful consultation. One of the most powerful tools the consultant has is his or her own awareness. Third, there are a multitude of roles for the internal consultant, and no one role is sufficient for all situations. In one setting the consultant will want to be very directive, while in another setting the consultant will want the client to be directive.

In this chapter we have also provided a decision tree for responding to the question: What is the most important role for me to play in this specific consultation? Our goal has been to provide a tool that will enable the internal consultant to make decisions regarding the role to take.

II

The Process of
Internal Consulting

3

The Eight Stages in Internal Consulting

Consulting is a process that can extend over a few minutes or many years. Usually, however, consulting is not a one-interaction event but is rather a process involving several phases. Whether the consultation is five minutes or five years, we find it useful and important to follow a particular structure or plan. This plan is essentially a blueprint that moves the internal consultant effectively through the various key steps. Like a map, the process provides direction. Failure to follow the sequenced approach will often get the consultant into trouble because of missed information.

The consulting process is the "science" of consultation. This chapter contains a step-by-step walk-through — the "map" — of the process. It is most important for the person new to the internal consulting process. As with a person learning a new skill, the initial task is to learn the basics. The next transition is to move from the "science" or technique of the consulting process to the "art" of the process. Like the person who has mastered a skill, the consultant who has mastered the process now has the option to be creative in her or his exploration of the process. Consultation now becomes an art form.

The next few chapters are about the consulting process. In Chapters One and Two we discussed the role of the internal consultant. This chapter provides the framework for the internal consultant's work.

Perhaps a useful place to begin is with the following story. Several years ago we set out to do an internal consulting job. The director of the laboratory asked us to do a team-building session with his supervisors. We spent a few minutes listening to the director's analysis of what he needed. Without much further planning, we set off to do the team-building event, and an event it was. The more we got into the venture, the more we realized that we had not done our homework sufficiently. For example, in the middle of the event we found that the views of the director and the supervisors were not even remotely similar. We completed the session, but we relearned a very basic lesson — do the homework.

Now, when we refer to that session, we say that it was like walking out and shooting a shotgun into the sky hoping that a duck will fly through. The shotgun approach will work occasionally. However, we recommend a much more targeted approach.

Successful internal consulting is not an accident. It is the result of a well-planned and thought-through process.

Learning from External Consultants

Before we get into our general model for internal consulting, we want to return once more to the discussion in Chapter One regarding external and internal consultants. We find that, as internal consultants, we can learn a good deal from external consultants. Perhaps one of the most basic learnings has to do with how the external consultant goes about her or his business.

Try this exercise. Think for a moment about consultants you have known and respected. What was it about their approach or style that was attractive to you? What were the behaviors that you noted?

Here are some of our responses to the question; compare them with yours. One of the major qualities of successful external consultants is that they are acutely aware of the consulting process and are very professional in their approach and attitude. They do not take their clients for granted or assume that their clients have no other options. Their professionalism includes timeliness, manner of dress, communication skills, non-

The Eight Stages in Internal Consulting

judgmental attitude, flexibility, enthusiasm, and energy. If the external consultant desires a contract with a client, she or he will be certain to use an approach that involves a step-by-step contracting process and communicates to the client that the consultant knows what she or he is doing. A major key is that the external consultant is willing to say "no" to a potential client. Saying "no" is an important topic that we will discuss further later in this chapter.

To summarize, the external consultant:

- communicates professionalism through behaviors and thought
- brings a well-thought-through process to the client, that is, has a procedure for how to go about the consulting process
- brings an excitement and can-do attitude to settings that may be experiencing "stuckness"

In the world of the internal consultant, the situation is a little different. The approach is often not as polished. The dress is often a little more informal. The flexibility is often not as great. Even the handouts and audiovisual (AV) materials are not quite the quality of those the external consultant would use. Contracts, if used at all, are usually verbal and brief. In our experience, internal consultants frequently are more informal, paying less attention to the details of the consulting process than external consultants. Internal consultants have more of a tendency to take their work for granted.

The Consulting Process

We have referred a good deal thus far to the consulting process. The remainder of this chapter provides an overview of the parts of the consulting process model. Each aspect of the model will be discussed in detail in a later chapter. The model contains the following parts:

1. Precontracting
2. Contracting

Figure 12. Nolan Model.

Initial client contact

Informal / Formal

Secondary / Primary

Proactive / Reactive

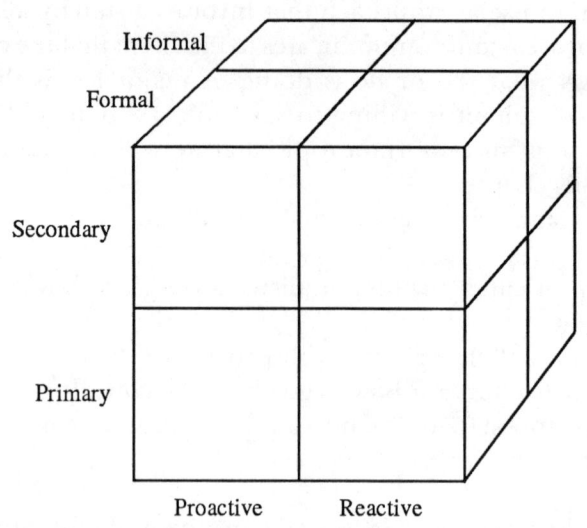

Source: Nolan, 1982. Copyright © 1982 by Tim Nolan, Ph.D. Used with permission.

3. Data collection
4. Data analysis
5. Presentation
6. Action planning
7. Evaluation
8. Termination

Step 1: Precontracting. The consultation process begins with an initial contact with a client. Nolan (1982) has developed a model for the initial client contact (see Figure 12). The model has the following characteristics:

1. *Proactive.* The internal consultant initiates the contact with the client group. Perhaps the internal consultant has heard that some problems are brewing or perhaps simply makes it a point to visit client groups on a regular basis. The important point is that the contact is initiated by the consultant.

2. *Reactive.* The initial contact comes about as a result of

The Eight Stages in Internal Consulting

someone else's initiation or activity. The internal consultant is brought in at some point by someone else. For example, we were recently asked to consult with a third party by the third party's boss. The contact came about because of another person's activity.

3. *Formal.* The initial contact is a structured meeting between the client and the internal consultant ("I would like to meet with you on the twenty-ninth at eight o'clock"). There has been planning, and contact is intentional.

4. *Informal.* The initial contact is not a structured event of some type between the consultant and the client. For example, you might meet someone for coffee to have an informal discussion and have that individual turn into a client.

5. *Primary.* The initial contact is face to face. You have a chance to talk directly with the client and to observe the client's verbal and nonverbal behaviors.

6. *Secondary.* The initial contact is made in an impersonal way. For example, it might be by memo, or someone might tell you that so and so wants to talk with you about a particular issue.

Nolan's discussion of the initial contact and the possibilities for that contact become very useful. Why? Frequently, the initial contact sets the stage for what will follow. Some consultants believe that the first two minutes of a relationship set the tone for the total relationship. Think about that for a moment. Do you recall the experience of meeting someone and deciding almost immediately that that person would be a "thorn in the side" or a close friend? The point is that we need to pay attention to those first few minutes because they can set the tone for the rest of the relationship.

The same is true of the initial contact with a possible client. Impressions are being formed, and basic information, both verbal and nonverbal, is being exchanged. The better information you have as an internal consultant, the better you will be able to respond to the client.

Think about the Nolan model and your experience. Try to remember some examples from your experience of each type of contact (proactive, reactive, formal, informal, primary, and secondary).

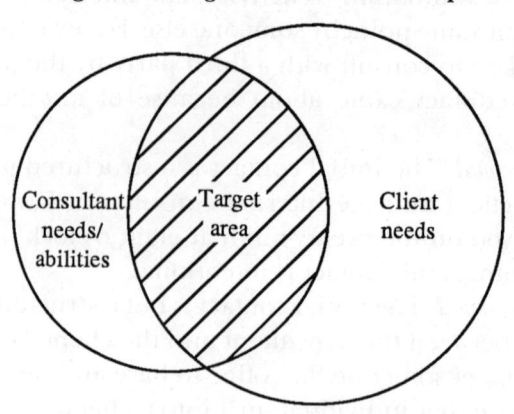

Figure 13. Target Area: Needs Overlap.

[Venn diagram: Consultant needs/abilities | Target area | Client needs]

We have found that the informal and the unplanned discussions are frequently the initial contact with a client. It is not unusual to have a client seek us out in an informal setting. In fact, we like to make ourselves available for unplanned, informal contacts. For example, after a management development program, it is not unusual to have several persons talk to us about "some things they have been thinking about."

We prefer our initial client contact to be in person in either a formal or an informal setting. The goal of this time is to see if there is enough common ground with the client to continue to the next step. In some of the literature, this time is referred to as a time of "scouting," and that literally is what is going on (see Figure 13).

Why is this time so important? Again, the first few minutes of a helper-helpee relationship will frequently set the tone for the rest of the relationship. If the relationship gets off to a rocky start, that will carry over to the rest of the relationship. One of the standard assumptions that we work from is that all behavior is data. How the first contact is made is data. If the client is late for a series of meetings, that is data that we need to consider. If the client is distrustful of us, that is data. All client behavior is data, and the early interactions provide useful initial data.

In addition to the relationship, this is the internal consul-

The Eight Stages in Internal Consulting 61

tant's first decision point. The problem is how to get enough information to decide whether or not to continue in the consulting process.

The key for this time is a decision regarding the next steps. The internal consultant is considering: "Is this something that I believe I can do? Do I have the skills to do it? Are there other agendas that are coming into play? Are there political considerations that I need to think about? Is the client leveling with me at this point? Are the right players involved in the discussion? Who is not here that needs to be here?" and many more questions.

The internal consultant needs to be able to say yes or no to continuation of the process. The internal consultant who cannot say no is in serious trouble, because she or he becomes locked into every issue that comes along. This will mean an ineffective use of the internal consultant's time and resources.

Step 2: Contracting: Clarifying Tasks and Relationships. Assuming that we have decided that we can be useful for the client and that we want to proceed, the time has come for entering into a formal contracting process that involves defining the tasks and relationships.

The tasks are simply what things are to be done by whom and by what time. It means defining what the finished product will look like. If the task is problem solving, the steps of how that will happen are identified and mapped out.

The relationships concern the client's expectations for the internal consultant and the internal consultant's expectations for the client. The roles are defined at this point. Does the client expect the internal consultant to be a director, or does the client want the internal consultant to be more of a facilitator? What about the internal consultant? Does the internal consultant want the client to take a lead in the meetings? Or does the internal consultant want to take the lead?

Contracting is a time of defining the specific steps in the consultation process. The key decision of contracting is once again: Do we have enough in common to continue this relationship? Precontracting is like a first date. At the end of precontracting is a decision of whether to date again. Contracting is like arriving at the decision to continue.

Step 3: Data Collection. When the decision is that client and consultant have enough in common to continue, it is time to collect whatever data are needed to arrive at needed decisions.

There are numerous data collection methods. The primary methods include questionnaires, interviews, and observations. The pros and cons of these methods will be discussed in a later chapter.

The key decisions that must be made at this time are what information is needed, who must be involved in the decision-making process, and what the most effective method of collecting the information is.

Step 4: Data Analysis. After the data have been collected comes the time of data analysis. What is the best way to do the analysis of the data? How do we turn the data into useful decision-making information?

Data that are qualitative (for example, clients' comments on a question) or quantitative (for example, numeric responses to a question) may need analysis. It is very important that the internal consultant be sensitive to the nature of the data—or, as we describe it, let the problem do the talking (Ulschak, 1978, pp. 148–153).

Step 5: Presentation. Somewhere in the process there will be a time of data presentation. The internal consultant needs to make decisions regarding the best way to communicate the collected data and to whom. Whether those data are presented to an individual or to a group, the data need to be communicated and discussed.

Client participation in the response to the data is very important. Regardless of the role in which the consultant might be, she or he should use the client as a final judge of whether or not the data fit. If the client does not agree with the outcomes, the consultant needs to reevaluate. This is another decision

The Eight Stages in Internal Consulting 63

point. At minimum, during this time, the consultant should ask the client to comment on how he or she agrees with the data.

Step 6: Action Planning. This step grows out of step 5 and sometimes is included as part of step 5. The consultant has the data and now must decide what steps need to be taken by whom and when, the desired outcomes, and under what conditions. By this time action planning is simple and straightforward. All the work has been done in the previous steps and now comes to fruition. The action plan may be as simple as a verbal agreement on next steps or as complex as a detailed computer-driven project plan.

Step 7: Evaluation. The final step is asking whether we got done what we needed to and whether we did it in a manner that used our resources effectively and efficiently.

The key evaluation question is: Did we get done what needed to get done? If some parts are unfinished or incomplete, our task is to decide if we need to do more work with them. Our options are to:

1. Declare the project over and a success.
2. Declare parts of the project a success and continue to work on the remainder of the project. This means recycling back to the contracting stage of the consultation.
3. Do an autopsy. The project was not a success, but our decision is to go no further with it.

If we have followed the steps to this point, the evaluation is a simple process. The other steps provide the data for the evaluation.

Step 8: Termination. The final step is termination. When to terminate a project can become an issue for the internal consultant because the internal consultant remains in the organization. Whether the project was an outstanding success or a failure, the internal consultant and the client need a time to complete separation. Remember—the consultation is not just an exchange of information. In every consultation there will be some degree of relationship, and termination means an ending of that relationship.

Termination might simply be a discussion where the internal consultant says, "I enjoyed working with you." It may be a significant time of discussing and rehashing the journey of the relationship. Termination is a time of parting, and it needs a degree of intentionality.

Reflections on the Model

Like all models, the usefulness of this one lies in its ability to provide a road map for how the consultation should flow. If you follow the process completely, you will probably be successful in your internal consultant work. You will have touched all the bases. However, for various reasons, many times you will not follow the process through completely. You will leave out some steps or bypass them. In this way, the process is situational—you will adapt the process to your situation. For example, you may find that the contracting process itself is sufficient for the consultation. At the end of contracting the client may repeat that he or she is back on track and does not need to go further, or you may find that partway through the consultation you need to recontract. Conditions change, and so will the contract.

In the next several chapters we will discuss these steps in detail and identify skills needed for each.

We will close this chapter with three examples of the consulting process.

Example 1: A Computer Program

This first example was chosen because it provides a quick overview of the internal consulting process.

Initial Meeting. The initial meeting was a hallway discussion in which an HR person (client) was asking a number of questions regarding staffing.

The Eight Stages in Internal Consulting

Client: By the way, we have a need for a way to get at the exit interview material we are collecting. Right now it is collected, but we really cannot use it in any effective way. Would you be willing to do some work on it?

Consultant: Sounds like it could be an interesting project. Right now I am busy with a number of other projects, but in a couple of weeks I would be able to do some work on it. I would want to talk more with you to see if it is something that I can do or if it is something for which you would want to get another person.

Client: Sounds good. I will give you a call in a couple of weeks.

Contracting. The contracting was in a formal meeting set up by the client to discuss the development of a computer program for an area of human resources.

Client: I am glad we were able to get our busy schedules together and to meet to discuss the exit interviews. We currently gather the data, but we do not have an effective report system. We decided since we are early into it that we would like to get it computerized, and that is where your name came up. We know that you are interested in computers and do lots of work in this area.

Consultant: I am certainly interested in the project, and I have a number of questions. Some of the questions have to do with the outcomes you are looking for, and other questions focus for me what your expectations are.

First, for what outcomes are you looking?

Client: We want a report that will summarize the responses to the exit interview questionnaires that we can then distribute to administration.

Consultant: Let's imagine for a moment that you have that report in front of you. When you look at it, what do

	you see? What is the format? How is it laid out? Is it for a specific department or a specific time frame?
Client:	Good questions. Yes, it would be a report that could be broken down by department and for specific time frames. It would also show a frequency count for each question, and what percent that... (The client continues to identify the outcomes for the project. The internal consultant continues to clarify what the client needs. One of the important things happening is that the internal consultant is also checking out if he has the skills to do this specific job.)
Consultant:	Good. I think that I have a good understanding of the outcomes. Let's take a few minutes to talk about time frames. With what kind of time frames are you working? Is there any urgency here about which I need to know?
Client:	In two months I need to have this ready for my boss. Is two months sufficient for your schedule?
Consultant:	Two months should be fine for this project. However, what I would like to do is take a couple of days and explore the project a bit more. How about if I drop off a one-page proposal in two days that summarizes my understanding of the project and what I can deliver and by when?
Client:	Sounds fine to me.
Consultant:	Excellent. One last question. I see my role here as providing you with a program. I would like to essentially work on my own until I have it completely drafted and then show it to you. Do you want more frequent contact than that? Or does that sound fine?
Client:	No, I would like you to follow the guidelines, but we do not have to have frequent meetings...

Data Collection. The internal consultant gets copies of the exit interview form and talks to the person who presently is

The Eight Stages in Internal Consulting

responsible for questionnaire collection to find out how that person feels about the questionnaire.

Data Analysis. The internal consultant summarizes the material from the other discussions and begins to think about how much time each step will take.

Presentation. The internal consultant is now to meet with the client once more and present a one-page written summation of the project with time lines.

Consultant: Here is my proposal. I will be able to have the project done in ten weeks. I recognize that means it will be two weeks later than you would like, but my other commitments are such that it will take that long. I have listed out each task and how long it will take for me to do. I have also listed out resources that I will need from you. For example, I will need you to provide me with a secretary to enter data, and that will take three to four hours.

Client: The secretarial time should not be a problem. However, the ten weeks is. If I were to provide you with more help, could you meet the eight-week deadline? (Now some negotiation begins between the client and the internal consultant. This continues, and an agreement is finally reached.)

Action Plan. The previous step incorporated the action plan, so now the action steps are implemented.

Evaluation. Because of the effective contracting, the evaluation process is simple. It asks whether the computer program is doing what the client wants.

Consultant: We have finished the work, and here is the draft report. The bugs are out of the system, and the only question is if this report is sufficient for you.

Client: It looks excellent. This is more than I had hoped for. One question: How easy would it be to add more employee information to this report?

Consultant: To add information that is not on the questionnaire would be another complete project. We would need to see it as a new project. My suggestion is that you try this for six to eight months and then see what might be changed.

Client: Agreed.

Termination.

Client: Let's get to together for coffee and a donut—on me. You have done an excellent job, and I want to let you know it.

Consultant: Sounds good. Let's take some time to just review this project and see what we might have done differently if we were starting over from scratch.

Example 2: Operating Room Manual

One of the privileges of writing these scenarios is that we get to set them up any way we like. Most consultations, however, do not go this smoothly. Our next example is that of a contracting process that has gone astray.

The education department was requested by the operating room department to work with them on the development of a manual for an extensive operating room program. Development of an operating room manual was one organizational objective. The first phase was to design a manual that would be used in the operating room program.

The two key players in the project were the nursing director of the operating room and the oncology nurse consultant (education department).

Contracting. The initial meeting took place to discuss the typing of the manual.

The Eight Stages in Internal Consulting 69

Client (nursing director): I called this meeting to discuss the development of the operating room nursing program. As you know, we will be doing the bulk of the development, and what we need is to have someone do the editing and take care of the actual publication.

Consultant: We are very interested in facilitating the project. I have a few questions to ask regarding time frames and the amount of typing required.

Client: It looks like there will be ten sections, six of which are drafted, and there are currently about two hundred pages. I will need the first six chapters over the next two months, and I'll continue to give you the rest as it gets developed.

Consultant: As you're aware, our secretarial resources are scarce. However, we will take on this typing project and work with you on it. When will you be getting the material to us? . . .

This brief encounter is a good example of moving too quickly to be pleasing to a client group. Specific information regarding the project was not obtained. For example, specific time frames were not developed, what the end product should look like was not discussed, how many drafts were expected did not enter into the discussion, and how the information was going to be given to the education department (for example, handwritten notes versus typed notes, and so on) was not clarified. There was no formally written contract comprising all the necessary project details. Tasks and relationships were not defined. The result was a later series of meetings in which the client expressed dissatisfaction with us and we expressed dissatisfaction with the client.

Data Collection. The decision was that we would continue and take on the typing of the manual. Essentially, our data collection was receiving the draft of the first six chapters. This was a "surprise" for us, as the material was not in a form that could be easily typed or understood. For example, the handwriting was illegible, there was no similar structure of headings, the content format varied from one chapter to the next since they were written by various authors, and so on.

At this time the oncology consultant went back to discuss the situation with the director. Some changes were made, and we continued typing and editing the manual as best we could. This continued for several weeks. We then started to get major redrafts of the first several chapters. A new clinical specialist with specific responsibility to complete the manual had been hired into the operating room. Her assessment was that it needed to be completely redone.

At this point we felt that we were almost starting over because of the massive revisions. Then we received additional chapters, another thing we had not discussed in contracting.

We called a meeting at which we discussed our findings and problems. We presented our plan of action, which was to complete the two chapters on which we were working. We would not be able to accept any other redrafts or additional chapters to be typed.

The discussion was brief, and both sides left the meeting with hard feelings. This was a situation that needed mending and would take some time to correct.

The above is a good example of the consulting process not being used to its fullest with the result of much wasted time.

Example 3: Team Building

The initial contact was via a telephone call from a nursing director to the consultant. The nursing director requested a meeting to discuss a problem that she was having with one of her areas. She reported that there was a serious team issue and wanted to meet with the consultant in the next day or so.

Contracting.

Consultant: How can I be useful for you? It sounded over the phone like you were in a crisis of some type.
Client: You are right there. Recently, several staff have come to me regarding their supervisor. They feel

The Eight Stages in Internal Consulting

	like she is just not there for them. They are discouraged and upset with the organization for not being more responsive to them. I need your help in thinking through this issue.
Consultant:	Okay. Let me ask a couple of questions. First, how serious a problem do you think it is? If nothing were done, what would the problem look like in three months?
Client:	That's easy. In three months, I would be searching for new staff. I will be having significant turnover.
Consultant:	So, it sounds as if this is something that you see needing to be addressed immediately.
Client:	Correct. I would like to be able to demonstrate that we are moving ahead to try and correct the situation.
Consultant:	One question that I have is about your relationship with the supervisor. Have you talked with her about this? Do you believe that she is a salvageable person?
Client:	Yes, we have talked, and she wants to do whatever is needed to improve the situation. She is new to supervision and needs to develop as a supervisor. I would like us to involve her in the next meeting so that she can get on board with us.
Consultant:	Excellent. Here is how I normally like to work in this kind of setting. First, I would like to do a number of interviews with staff in your area. These will take thirty to forty minutes, and I will be getting from them the issues that the staff see within the work team. Next, I will take those interviews and summarize them for a general meeting of the staff where the themes will be discussed and action planning will take place. Of course, I will respect confidences and will not report specific comments by specific individuals.

(The next meetings consisted of the director, the supervisor, and the consultant.)

Consultant: In the last meeting I discussed how I like to work, and I know the two of you have discussed that. Do you have any questions?

Client: The one question that came up as we talked is the time line for this project. How soon could we get it under way, and how long would it take?

Consultant: I could begin in about two weeks. It takes about two weeks to complete the interviews, another week to do the analysis, and I should be ready to present the results in about three weeks.

Client: Good. Let's begin.

Consultant: The first question is how we manage the process. We need to decide the best process for letting the staff know what will be happening and why. Our goal is to get their full cooperation. Mr. Supervisor, when do you have your next meeting?

(A meeting is set with staff to discuss the process, the reason, and the expected outcomes.)

Data Collection. Data collection consisted of interviews of key staff by the consultant. The questions concerned what was going right, what was not working, and what needed to happen to correct the items that were not working.

Data Analysis. The consultant then did a listing of the key themes that came out during the interviews. Individuals' comments were kept confidential.

Presentation/Action Planning. Prior to the presentation of the material collected, the consultant had another meeting with the client and the supervisor.

Consultant: Here is how I would like to have this meeting run. First of all, I would like the supervisor to start the meeting and discuss why this process was set up and what our goals for it were. It is important that he be seen as the person in charge, since it is his

The Eight Stages in Internal Consulting 73

Client: work unit. My role will be to present the data and lead the group in a discussion of them. I would like the supervisor to then work with me as we discuss action steps. How does that sound?
Client: What about my role?
Consultant: Good question. I would like you to make an opening statement that you see these kind of meetings as valuable and you are pleased that this work unit is doing it. Then, I would like you to spend your time listening...

(The meeting proceeded according to plan. The outcome was a specific action plan that listed steps to be taken by whom and when.)

Evaluation. (Three weeks later, the consultant made an informal call to the client to find out the status of the project.)

Consultant: I wanted to check back with you to see how things are going. How are things on the unit?
Client: Well, the crisis has certainly eased. There are still a number of problems, but the general sense is that there is movement on the problems...

Summary

This chapter has provided an overview of the consulting process. Our purpose has been to identify the steps in the process. These steps are precontracting, contracting, data collection, data analysis, presentation, action planning, evaluation, and termination. Again, our belief is that the steps are important for the internal consultant to use as a guide to provide direction in thinking through a consultation process.

The next several chapters will take the steps we have described and discuss them in detail.

4

Establishing an Effective Relationship with the Client

Many organizations today focus much energy and money into ensuring consumer/client satisfaction. For many the question of *who* their clients are can be easily and readily answered. For others, it is not quite that easy. It is an impossible task to talk in terms of and work toward client satisfaction without first identifying who the client is. We discussed client identity in Chapter One.

It sounds simple enough. The person making the initial contact, the first step in the consulting model, is the client. Right? Well, *maybe* most of the time the person initiating the entry is indeed the client—but not always. Sometimes that person is the client's "messenger." Our role as consultant is to clearly and early identify the client.

The importance of identifying who the client is is illustrated in this experience of a friend's purchase of her first car. She decided to invite her brother along to get his opinions on the more mechanical end of the deal. She found the car of her dreams at the first car dealer. All was going well until the salesman came on the scene. He readily shook hands with and introduced himself to her brother, without as much as a glance in her direction. The salesman focused 100 percent of his attention and energies on the brother and ignored the woman's

Establishing an Effective Client Relationship 75

questions. After a few minutes of this interaction, the woman proceeded to give the salesman a detailed account of her impressions up to that point. "After all," she told him, "I am the one buying the car!" With that she turned on her heel and left the car of her dreams and a red-faced, open-mouthed salesman.

This story illustrates a valuable lesson for all consultants. Much time and energy can go into impressing the wrong person at the expense of insulting the client. *Know your client.*

Argyris (1973, p. 31) suggests that the role of the interventionist (what we call the internal consultant) in a system is to do three things: (1) generate valid and useful information, (2) create conditions for the clients to make free and informed choices, and (3) help clients develop internal commitments to choices.

There are many ways to discuss the purpose of contracting. Argyris's three points summarize it nicely. First, the purpose is to generate information that is both valid and useful for the client. It is not unusual, in this day of computers, to be able to generate volumes of data not useful for the client.

Many questions need to be answered. What are valid data? What really is the client's problem? How did the problem start? What keeps it a problem? How is the problem useful for the client (this is always a discussion starter)? What has the client tried to do in the past to address the problem? What will the situation look like in six months if the problem is not solved? What are the feelings of the client regarding the problem?

Second, the consultation needs to leave the client with informed choices. Note this choice of words. A key outcome of the consultation is that the client has a sense of options and is not locked in. A key role of the consultation is to help develop options.

Third, the consultation process needs to assist the client in developing commitment to the choices that get made. At times, the easy part of the consultation is getting the client to arrive at an option. The tough part is taking the next step and helping the client to answer the question: How do we get commitment to this particular option?

The key for the internal consultant during the contracting

process is to monitor these three elements. Is valid information being generated? Is the environment such that the client is developing a set of informed choices? What needs to happen to have the client become invested in the choices?

This chapter discusses what it takes to have an effective client relationship and effective contracting. Our belief is simple: the core of the effective consulting relationship is effective contracting.

What Is Contracting?

Contracting is the process of defining the tasks and the relationship between the client and the internal consultant. This may sound easy enough, but it can also be quite tricky. The goal of the contracting time is to define the task to be done and the roles to be performed by the client and the internal consultant. The internal consultant uses contracting to (1) clarify and define the relationship between the consultant and the client and (2) clarify with the client where the client is presently and where the client wants to get (defining tasks).

Contracting can be seen as both a process and a tool. As a process, contracting is used to explore and define the relationship between the internal consultant and the client. The client's wants and needs for services are detailed along with the range of services the internal consultant is willing and able to provide. This period is a time of deciding what the various parties involved want from each other, whether they have the ability and resources to provide what is wanted from the relationship, and whether they are willing to enter into the relationship. The essential process questions are:

1. What do we want and need from each other?
2. Do we have the ability and resources to do what is necessary?
3. Is each of us willing to move into this relationship?

However, contracting can also be used as a tool. The internal consultant may find that contracting as a tool is extremely valuable in many settings. Using contracting as a tool,

Establishing an Effective Client Relationship 77

the internal consultant can assist the client in identifying and evaluating the present situation and the desired future condition. The internal consultant then assists the client in selecting strategies that will accomplish the movement from the current conditions to the desired conditions. An example of this is the internal consultant who finds that her role is really to help the client think through options. The client may have an inner conflict that the internal consultant helps to surface and resolve. A major consultation is not needed as the solution is immediate.

One example is a setting in which we were involved where the client wanted to host a major meeting between two departments to work out "differences." However, in the process of using contracting as a tool, what surfaced was that the client had an internal conflict and was going to use the major meeting as the place to address this conflict. The client knew what he wanted to do, but he did not want to alienate others, and he knew that would happen if he proceeded with the action. We shifted the focus from the design of an interdepartmental meeting to the resolution of his inner conflict.

Essentially, contracting is a process of "horse trading" or marketplace bartering. It involves the parties' discussing what is wanted and who will do what when. A model that we like to use as a framework for discussing defining tasks and relationships is the "pinch model" (Scherer, 1975). The model is illustrated in Figure 14.

The pinch model begins with the beginning of some type of relationship. In our case, it is the relationship between the internal consultant and the client. Each party puts its best foot forward. They arrive at a mutual agreement regarding roles and relationships. The most productive time is the time when there is a sense of mutual agreement. However, as time passes, there are "pinches." Pinches are those small yet discernible sensations like: "I thought he was going to do that." "What did he mean by that statement to me?" "Who is going to do that part?" and the like. The pinch is a deviation from what was expected. The choice each time a pinch appears is to ignore it, hoping that it will go away, or to confront it.

It is best to confront pinches when you find yourself

Figure 14. Pinch Theory: A Model for Role Clarification and Negotiation.

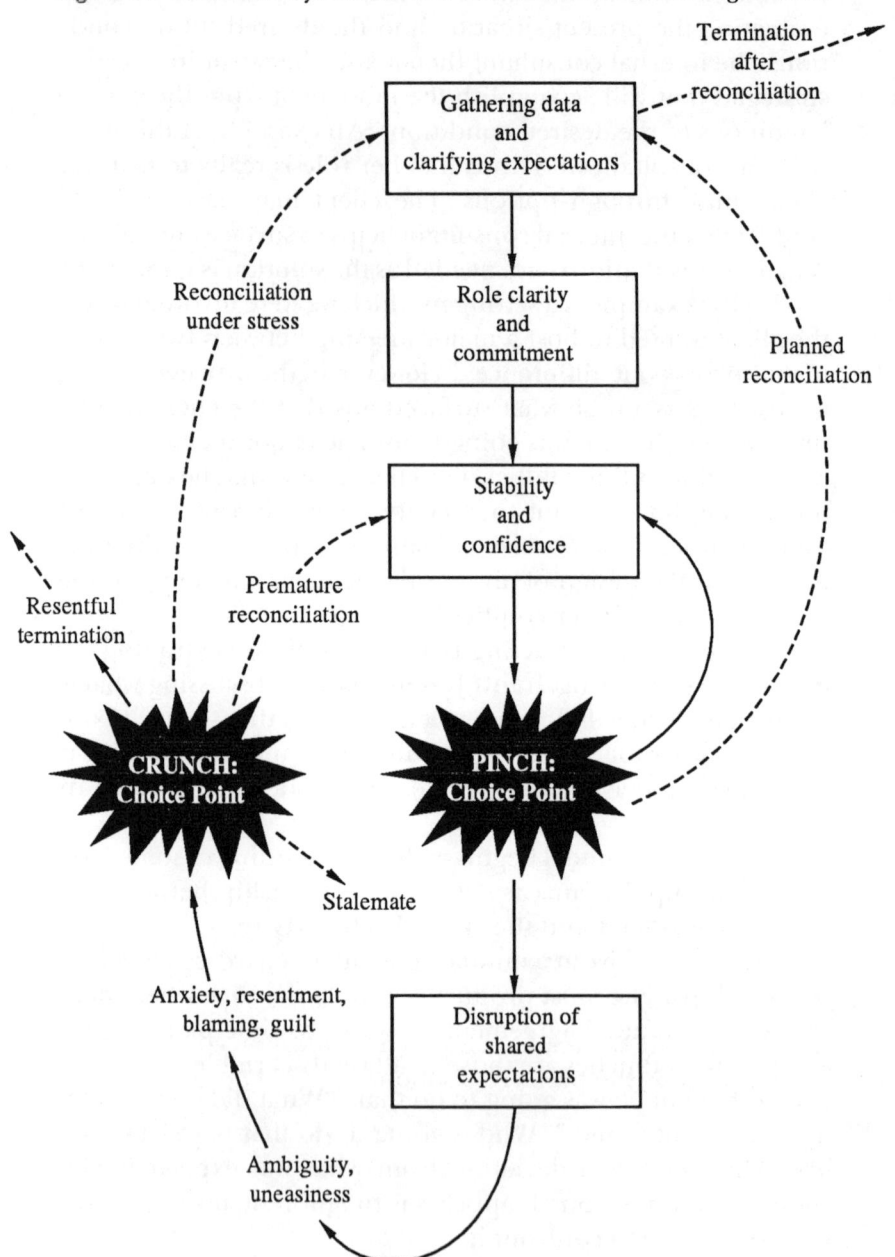

Source: Scherer, 1975. Reprinted by permission.

Establishing an Effective Client Relationship 79

thinking about them for more than a few minutes. If you find yourself thinking over and over, "Boy, did he let me down," that is a sign that the pinch should be confronted. The point of the confrontation is not to blame the other person but rather to go back to the initial agreement and renegotiate with the person.

The problem with ignoring pinches is that they have a tendency to collect and build. In the literature of transactional analysis, this is referred to as "stamp collecting." Those of you familiar with collecting green stamps with your groceries or other types of redemption stamps for products purchased will readily understand stamp collecting. Stamp collecting in the emotional sense goes something like this. As you go through your day or week, you collect emotional stamps. Someone says something to you. You smile, but you open your mental stamp book and paste in an "anger" stamp. The next person comments on the way you are dressed, and you place another "anger" stamp in the book. This continues until you reach the point where your book is full, and the next person who says something to you gets "dumped on." That person gets the whole load of your anger because of having made the statement that broke the camel's back. This is the essence of stamp collecting.

If you do not confront pinches, you might accumulate them until they become a "crunch." Then you have a serious relational problem. The options are to:

1. Leave the relationship. This can be a costly choice, since it means leaving everything behind.
2. Smooth over the relationship and try to start over. The problem to be watched here is back in the relationship.
3. Do nothing. This can readily lead to burnout.
4. Renegotiate the relationship. While this is time-consuming, it is usually the preferred option.

For contracting, the key dynamic of the pinch model is the concept that pinches are a given. There is no way to avoid them. They will occur. The only question, key for those in contracting, is how to manage them. Contracting is not a one-time deal. It needs feedback loops that update the contract. The pinches that are experienced need to be confronted.

Change is implicit in the use of contracting as a process and a tool. Contracting is a dynamic process that changes as conditions change. That is why feedback is so important. The parties to the contract need to keep one another informed as to changes that impact the contract.

Contracting in the realm of internal consulting has a different quality than that of external consulting. The internal consultant never has a clean slate with the client. The client may be favorably or unfavorably predisposed to the internal consultant. Remember our earlier comments regarding internal and external consultants. The internal consultant is part of the family and is a known commodity.

What does this mean? It means that each party brings to the consultation something of a history with the other. For the internal consultant, this may mean he or she will approach the client with less intentionality than he or she would as an external consultant. For example, the internal consultant might not allow himself or herself the luxury of saying no, or he or she may already have the inside story from others in the organization. Such things can influence the course of the consultation and create a messy relationship. Our goal is to keep the relationship as clean as possible so that the work of the consultation can get done effectively.

A Process of Defining the Tasks and Relationships

The intent of contracting is to clarify what needs to be done and by whom. The first part of contracting is ensuring that parties understand the task to be done. This can happen in several ways.

The first way to define the task is to simply ask the client what needs to happen. In some settings the client is clear about this, and the task is readily defined. The client has been living with the problem and knows it well. However, in most settings the client is not all that clear about what needs to happen. This means that the initial contact probably concerns a symptom

Establishing an Effective Client Relationship

rather than the cause. The client may not know the "real story" at this point or may not trust you with it.

Earlier we said that probably most clients do not know what the real problem is. This does not mean that we do not take seriously what the client tells us the problem is. It simply means that we do not stop with the client's statement. As the process outlined in the last chapter indicates, we start with the contract, but we continue beyond it. Much of the rest of the work is spent on clarifying and refining the contract.

The second way to define the task is to ask the client a set of questions to help the client clarify what the task is. We ask the client to focus on what it would be like if the problem were not a problem. What would things look like if everything were working well? What would the final printout look like? What would be going on? What would be happening? What this does is move the client from being stuck on "ain't it awful" to focusing on the desired state. In the process, the client centers on the desired outcome.

In the contracting concerning task, we typically like to ask questions such as:

1. What is the problem as you see it? Give as much detail as possible.
2. What are the immediate events that precipitated your contacting me? What has happened that is causing you to think about this problem?
3. What is the desired state? What would things look like if the problem were resolved?
4. What are some of the things keeping the problem a problem? What are some of the things preventing it from being resolved? Which of these is key, and how important is it?
5. What are some of the things moving the problem to resolution? What are some of the things that support resolution? Which of these is key, and how important is it?
6. If nothing were done to resolve the situation, what would be happening in six months?
7. When do you need to have it done?
8. Are there political implications of the task?

9. Have all the appropriate decision makers given the go-ahead on the project?
10. If you were describing the project to a colleague, what would you be saying about it?
11. What financial resources are available for the project, and who has what responsibilities?
12. What is your feeling regarding the project? Are you hopeful? Pessimistic?

Whenever possible, we try to be visual, using either a sheet of paper or a flip chart. For example, we like to draw a T chart with the left half of the sheet of paper or newsprint being the current conditions and the right half being the desired conditions. We then ask the client to make lists under each heading. We then ask, "How do we move from the current conditions to the desired conditions?" This is the work of the consultation.

The second part of the contracting is the relationship. Remember the earlier discussion regarding the basis for all behavior being perceptions. Each party in the relationship brings to the relationship a set of perceptions regarding self, the other person, and the problem that the relationship is built to solve. These sets of perceptions define the relationship's starting point.

The set of perceptions brought to the contracting will either facilitate the contracting and accomplishment of the purpose of the contracting session, or it will impede the accomplishment. Please note that talking about the relationship does not mean that either party needs to like the other party. While liking working with another person certainly makes the work more enjoyable, it is not always necessary. The key criterion is a willingness to keep clear with one another regarding purpose, role, and commitment.

When we talk about roles, we are talking about how the internal consultant and the client will relate to each other during the project. There should be discussion about which role for the internal consultant will be the most effective: director, counselor, facilitator, or delegator. The client and internal consultant

Establishing an Effective Client Relationship

need to identify what they see in terms of roles. They also need to agree about how a role change will happen.

Three very important understandings regarding the internal consultant–client relationship grow out of the work of Schutz (1984). Schutz identified three behaviors as foundational in relationships. The first behavior is termed *inclusion* and concerns the degree of inclusion each party desires. Some clients will want to know everything about the project that is going on. They have a high need for inclusion. If they are not included, they will cause trouble. For example, we have a client to whom we write a memo about almost everything because that client has a high need for inclusion and will create trouble if feeling left out. There will be others in the organization who are not immediately involved in the project but will want to know what is going on. Again, this signals a high inclusion need. In contrast, there will be others in the organization who will want not to see you until the project is completed. These people have a low need to be included. Still others will want to be included at critical points in the project. One important discussion with the client, then, is regarding the amount of inclusion he or she desires. One of the tasks of the consultant is to explore with the client the amount of inclusion that both need.

The second behavior is that of *control*. The person with control is the one who calls the shots. Again, some clients will want to control what is happening, which will be obvious to you in the first few minutes since they will control the setting. They will say they want this and this and this from you by this date and will tell you what to do and how to do it. Other clients will want you to be in control of the setting. They will want you to take the director role. Again, what is important is that you and the client arrive at some agreement regarding the degree of control the client and you each want.

The third behavior is *openness*. Openness is the degree of closeness that you and the client want. Some internal consultants like to get close to their clients, and others do not. Again, what is important is that you and the client agree on the degree of closeness.

With all three behaviors, the main issue is that there be time to discuss the relationship and what is expected from it. A mismatch on these dimensions can cause the work of the relationship, that is, the task, to abort. For example, if you want more openness from the client than the client is willing to give, and the client wants to control more than you are willing to be controlled, the relationship can be off to a rocky start.

There are two aspects for each of the dimensions of inclusion, control, and openness. The first aspect is how much of each participants want to receive. The second aspect is how much participants want to give. One aspect relates to the reception and the other to the giving. The problem is when there is a mismatch between the two.

The relationship side of contracting is frequently overlooked because at times it is more difficult to get at. For example, in your day-to-day work, you work with others whom you already know, and spending time on a relationship with them appears wasteful, yet the relationships are the foundation on which the rest of the consultation rests.

Here are some of the questions that may be used in defining a relationship with a client:

1. What do you want from me? How can I be of most use to you in this process?
2. How much do you want me to take the lead? When do you want to take the lead?
3. How much do you want to be included in the process?
4. What is expected of me with regard to openness? How open do I need to be in this relationship? How open will the client be with me in this relationship?
5. How would you like me to relate to you? What would you like for me not to do?

In addition to these relationship questions, the internal consultant needs to ask questions of himself or herself such as:

1. Is this a task that I am competent to do?
2. Is this a task that I can fit within my time priorities and commitments?

Establishing an Effective Client Relationship

Figure 15. CPR + F Model.

```
    ┌──────────────┐◄─────────────┐
    │  Commitment  │              │
    └──────┬───────┘              │
           ▲                      │
           ▼                      │
    ┌──────────────┐      ┌───────────────┐
    │   Purpose    │◄─────│   Feedback    │
    └──────┬───────┘      └───────────────┘
           ▲                      │
           ▼                      │
    ┌──────────────┐              │
    │     Role     │◄─────────────┘
    └──────────────┘
```

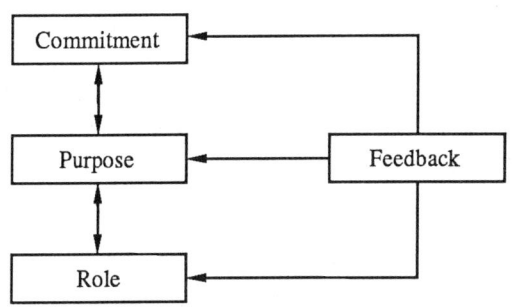

Source: Ulschak, 1989.

3. What is the down side of not doing this task? What is the down side of doing the task?
4. Are there any legal or ethical issues involved that need to be addressed?
5. What might be some ways that I might sabotage the task or relationship?

Contracting, then, is designed to define the task and the relationship. Successful contracting is the foundation of a successful project.

Effective Consultant-Client Relations: CPR + F Model

This chapter is about building effective consultant-client relationships through contracting. Take a few moments and think about effective relationships that you have had with consultants and clients and what the key elements of those relationships were.

We find that an effective internal consultant–client relationship can be built around the CPR + F model, shown in Figure 15 (Ulschak, 1989). Each element of the model will be discussed in detail.

1. *Purpose.* The client and the internal consultant both need to have a clear sense of the consultation's purpose. Without a common purpose the consultation is like a river overflowing its

banks—it may have lots of energy, but the energy is scattered and undirected. There is nothing quite as defeating or wearing as having excitement and energy but being directionless (purposeless). In our experience, a lack of clear purpose is one of the four key major reasons why a consultation fails.

A key function of contracting is defining a common purpose. A lack of common purpose will bring the consult to its knees. Defining purpose is another way of talking about defining task.

2. *Roles.* Both the client and the internal consultant need to have a clear sense of their own roles and the roles of other involved parties. The parties involved know who is responsible for what.

The second most common failing of the contracting process and the consultation process is a lack of clear definition of roles. It is hard to keep a common purpose if participants have questions about their roles or about who will do what when. Just as lack of purpose will confuse and depower a consultation, a lack of role agreement and clarity will also. Think about a time when you have been in a situation with a lack of role clarity. Most often the experience is one of confusion and frustration.

3. *Commitment.* The level of commitment to purpose and value of each party should be about the same, from medium high to high. We call this the "Goldilocks approach": the levels of commitment are not too hot, not too cold, but just right. Low levels of commitment generally mean that the project is not significant at this time, and sustained high levels of commitment can lead to burnout if they are consistent and long term.

Another term that is used for commitment is *investment* (Maehr and Braskamp, 1986). What is the client's investment in the consultation, and what is the consultant's investment? We were recently in a consultation where the client perceived an immediate problem and had great investment, but the consultant saw it as a minor problem and had minimum investment. Needless to say, there was significant conflict between the two.

Ideally, both parties should have about the same level of commitment. If they do not, it is important that they discuss the

Establishing an Effective Client Relationship

levels of investment and arrive at common understandings and agreement regarding each other's investment.

In our experience, the third area of failure of a consultation has to do with a lack of commitment.

4. *Feedback*. Mechanisms should be in place for providing feedback between the internal consultant and the client. This means that throughout the project, information is exchanged back and forth, allowing the project to correct its course.

Feedback is a given within the consultation process. Without feedback, the best contracting is for nothing. The reason: conditions change from day to day and week to week. This is especially true in health care. Without feedback loops, the consultant and client can easily get out of touch. The effective relationship is one that has periodic checkout loops. A lack of feedback is the fourth major reason why consultations fail.

The effective consulting relationship has all four of these components. Contracting is the time of defining each component.

We have not yet discussed the actual task accomplishment, which is what the relationship is all about. The purpose of the consult is to get something done. However, we found that at times premature outcome focus can actually get in the way of a successful consultation. For example, we have seen cases where the task focus was premature and, without the corrective mechanisms, led to a waste of resources. Consequently, we focus on the process that leads to the desired outcomes. Our belief: the effective process will lead to successful outcomes.

CPR + F Model: Contracting Framework

The CPR + F model is a specific framework for viewing the contracting process. This model focuses on four aspects of the contracting process. Again, they are (1) commitment of the parties involved, (2) purpose of the involvement, (3) roles of the parties involved, and (4) feedback loops.

The CPR + F model needs to be reviewed in light of the client and the internal consultant. It is not a tool just to review the client. When these four elements are adequately addressed in the contracting process, the consulting process will flow smoothly.

Commitment refers to the investment that the client and the consultant have in the task. How invested are they in this consultation? It is important to identify the degree of commitment that the client has to the task early in the consultation. Is the task one that someone else has said needs to be addressed, or one that the client has determined needs to be addressed? A key is to understand the client's degree of investment in the activity of the consultation.

In a recent consulting event, we found that we had grossly underestimated the client's degree of investment. We ended up spending hours and hours of time and investment in the project only to find that the client had nearly forgotten that we were even working on it. Our investment was high, but the initial client investment was low. The client should have a greater energy involvement in the project than the internal consultant. If the internal consultant is investing more than the client, something needs to be evaluated in the relationship.

Commitment relates not just to the client but also to the internal consultant. What is the internal consultant's level of commitment to the project? This is an important question. If the internal consultant does not evaluate his or her level of commitment to the project, the result can be a client who is very involved in a project and an internal consultant who is working on it halfheartedly. Once again we have a mismatch problem. The internal consultant needs to be aware of his or her level of commitment and to include that in the discussion phase of the contracting process. A simple but effective question that we like to ask is: On a ten-point scale, with 10 being "highly committed to this project" and 1 being "this project is a waste," where are you? What would it take for you to give a score of 10?

Purpose has to do with what the task or project is. What are the desired outcomes? The client needs to define these with the internal consultant. The internal consultant has the role of clarifying the purpose with the client. Many of the questions discussed earlier relate to the purpose of the consultation. By

Establishing an Effective Client Relationship 89

the end of the contracting time, there should be a clear statement as to the consultation's purpose. The important point is that the contracting session leads to a definition of purpose or a plan for defining the purpose.

Roles are the third part of the equation. Again, these have been discussed in some detail. What is important is that the contracting session be a time of clarifying roles. One part of the role discussion concerns who will do what when. The other concerns expectations that the parties to the contract have for each other. "Here is what I want from you, and here is what I am willing to provide for you" — these are contracting statements. As we discussed earlier, role confusion will result in not only an ineffective contracting time but also an ineffective consultation.

The fourth component is *feedback*. A discussion of how feedback will be managed is needed as part of the contracting time. The first part of this is feedback on how the consultation is going. Are there problems with the data collection? What do we do if the action plan is ineffective? How will we know it? These are feedback questions. The other kind of feedback is feedback to the client regarding the problem, potential action steps, and so on.

In some settings feedback will be managed by regular meetings between the client and the consultant. In other settings feedback will happen only randomly. Whichever is the case, it is best to decide how feedback will be managed.

An important point with the CPR + F model is that four components influence each other. It is difficult to be invested in something if its purpose or your role is unclear. Once the purpose is clarified, however, the investment may grow rapidly. For example, the internal consultant may find that initially the client has very little investment in doing what is being requested. However, in the process of clarifying purpose, the client may become very invested. The four are dynamic and influence each other continually.

The CPR + F model, then, can be used as an effective tool for planning the contracting session and for evaluating the contracting session. For example, in planning the session, the consultant can use the model to ask questions like:

- *Purpose.* What is the purpose of the contracting session? What do I as the consultant want to get out of the session? What do I think the client wants out of the session?
- *Role.* How do I want to be during the session? Do I want to take a lead role in the discussion? Do I want to be an active listener? What role should I play?
- *Commitment.* How committed am I to working with this client? How committed am I to working with this project? What do I think is the client's level of commitment to the project?
- *Feedback.* Do we want to discuss the results of the meeting at the end of the meeting? Do we want to give ourselves feedback on how effective or ineffective we were in getting the purpose of the meeting met?

This kind of prior planning can be most useful in seeing that the meeting's work gets carried out. At the conclusion of the contracting session, the meeting needs to be summarized using the same format:

- *Purpose.* The purpose of the consultation will be to... We will know that purpose has been achieved when...
- *Role.* The role of each of the parties in the consultation will be to... The client will be responsible for getting the following items complete... The consultant will be responsible for the following items...
- *Commitment.* Our commitment levels to the project and to working together are... We will continue to monitor the commitment levels by...
- *Feedback.* In order to stay in touch during this process, we will meet... In addition, there will be a written update each...

The form in Exhibit 2 summarizes the premeeting planning.
The intent of the process is to keep clarity in the contracting. We believe that if we keep a clarity with the CPR + F model during the contracting time, an effective contract will result.

Establishing an Effective Client Relationship

Exhibit 2. Contracting: Applying the CPR + F Model.

Purpose
What is the client's purpose for this meeting?
What is your purpose for the meeting?
Is there any conflict between the two purposes?

Role
What is your role in the meeting?
What do you think the client wants your role to be?
What role do you want the client to play?

Commitment
Is this project something you want to do?
What is the client's level of commitment?
Are there any pitfalls in working with this client?
What is your history with this client?

Feedback
Do we want to discuss the results at the end of the meeting?
How open do we want to be with each other?

Considerations in Contracting

There are a number of considerations in contracting. These are (1) role of good information—truth telling, (2) contracting meeting, (3) written and verbal contracts, (4) defining confidentiality, and (5) involving the key decision makers.

1. *Contracting depends on good information.* Without good information the process grinds to a halt. Therefore, the primary question of any internal consultant is: To what degree is good information available here?

This means that "truth telling" is a critical element of the contracting time. Without it, the session becomes meaningless. Truth telling here does not mean "leveling" another person or disclosing secrets. It means simply stating what is true. It may be as simple as the internal consultant's saying, "My time commitments are such that I will not be able to get to this project for a few months" to a candid observation that the project looks like it is destined to fail. Thinking back in terms of the percept model, truth telling means telling what is true for the person talking. It means disclosing what that person is thinking and feeling about a project.

Typically we find responses like "truth tellers do not last long in this organization" or "no one else tells the truth, so why should I?" We are not talking about truth telling as a moral issue but about the fact that unless there is good information between you and the client, you will waste many hours and dollars.

The implication is that the internal consultant needs to be prepared to create conditions for a valid flow of truthful information between consultant and client. The consultant should ask the client for that flow of information early on in the consultation. This means that the consultant must be willing to share her or his view of the world with the client.

One last editorial comment. We believe that without good information or truth telling in an organization, the organization is not long for this world. When we have the opportunity to contact organizational "gurus," we like to ask, "What is the key learning that you have from your lifetime in working with organizations?" Without exception the responses have to do with valid information and truth telling, the lifeblood of the organization.

2. *The contracting meeting is a formal face-to-face meeting.* It is designed for one purpose: to bring together the internal consultant and the client to define the purpose and roles of the consultation. It may take a few minutes or several hours, depending on the nature of the consultation.

Contracting can also happen over the telephone and via memos. If the project is straightforward, these can be very effective. However, as projects increase in complexity, it becomes more necessary for contracting sessions to be face to face.

3. *Role of written contracts.* We believe strongly that a contracting session should be followed with a written understanding of the contracting session. The written contract should summarize the meeting, the agreed-on task, the roles involved, the time lines, and so on. Whatever is pertinent to the consultation should be part of the contract. Here is a sample memo follow-up to a contracting session:

The purpose of this letter is to summarize our meeting regardng the absenteeism study and action plan for your department. As I understand our agreement, the purpose of the study is to identify the causes of absenteeism in your specific department and then to recommend to you a minimum of two alternative courses of actions.

You are willing to let me access your records and to interview current employees regarding causes of absenteeism. I will provide you with a specific action plan for the project and will give you a full written report by the end of the project.

In addition, we agreed to meet weekly on the project until such time as the action plan is completed and approved. After that point in time, we will meet on a monthly basis. If there is any significant shift in the plan, we will meet to discuss the implications for the time line and the project.

I am excited with the project, and from our discussion it is clear that you are as well. I look forward to continued work with you.

If there are items that I have missed from our discussion, please let me know.

4. *Confidentiality is an ongoing issue with the contracting time.* Many times internal consulting deals with departmental "dirty linen," and the question "What is the role of confidentiality?" arises.

We have a simple response. Whatever goes on between you and the client is confidential unless it has legal or ethical implications or harm for the organization, in which case it is no longer confidential. For example, in the course of a consultation, if you find the client is involved in activities that put the organization at legal risk, your obligation is to the organization first and the client second.

If, however, you find that the client is engaged in activities that you feel are unethical, you should discuss this with the client. If those issues are significant enough to you, you may consider terminating the contract.

If the internal consultant believes that organizational harm will occur if the setting is not corrected, that consultant has a responsibility to let management know. Again, the ultimate client for the internal consultant is the organization, because that is to whom the consultant is ultimately responsible.

Outside of legal and ethical issues, the internal consultant only needs to answer why it is important for him or her to be discussing the client's project. Sometimes it may be appropriate to discuss a project—for example, if the internal consultant is stuck and needs external consult.

5. *Another consideration of the contracting process is whether the key actors are involved in the project thus far.* Is the person with whom you are having the discussion the appropriate person? Is this person the decision maker? Does he or she have the authority to authorize the project?

For example, in team building it is not unusual for a member of a department to say, "Boy, do we need team building. Will you come and work with us?" Our standard response is, "Of course. However, you need to have your manager talk to us. Set up a meeting with her and..."

Does the person you are dealing with have the organizational authority to commit resources to the project?

Contracting Pitfalls

There are a number of pitfalls in contracting. The first and most important pitfall is promising something that cannot be delivered. Many people are in health care and helping professions because they want to be useful and helpful. The internal consultant must be careful to resist this urge and not promise something that he or she cannot deliver.

One type of problem is that the consultant may promise something requiring a higher skill level than he or she possesses. The problem may also be that the consultant cannot deliver in a timely way. Internal consultants provide services, and they have a tendency to think, "If I say no to this, they may get someone else. Maybe they will even hire an outside person to come in and do this." The result is that the internal consultant may say yes to

Establishing an Effective Client Relationship

more things than his or her time will hold. Another problem might be taking on a high-risk project before an adequate cost-benefit analysis has been done.

Taking on projects that are inappropriate is another pitfall. Remember that for the internal consultant, the organization is the family. Perhaps a senior administrator asks for a project in a specific time frame. The first reaction of the internal consultant might be to please that decision maker rather than to evaluate the project. Also, the organizational reality is that the internal consultant will sometimes be responding to the political side of the organization. It is not unusual for a consultant to be asked to make a training intervention when the real issue is something other than training.

Another pitfall is taking on projects to which the internal consultant has a strong negative reaction. We believe that whenever a project is troubling you, you should take that seriously and listen to yourself. If you do not, there is a good chance that that troubled part will come out in another way. Frequently, the troubling part is an important consideration that you have overlooked. When you have that strong reaction, take time to explore it before agreeing to go further.

Another pitfall is not setting measurable desired outcomes. Not everything has to be measurable, but outcomes should be as measurable as possible. You never know if you have been successful if you have no type of measurement.

Last, and perhaps most important, a major pitfall is not taking the contracting process seriously enough and not asking needed questions. External consultants are usually much more attuned to contracting than internal consultants. Our goal is to increase the contracting skills of the internal consultant.

Contracting Example

The following is an example of telephone contracting.

Consultant: Good to hear from you. What can I help you with today?
Client: Well, I have been wanting to talk to you for some

time about your doing a talk to my group about the importance for them of guest relations. There are a couple of folks that really need that.

Consultant: What are some of the problems that you are having that cause you to think that this is needed? What are the signs and symptoms?

Client: Well, in the past two weeks, I have had three other departments take me aside and talk to me about problems they have had with my folks.

Consultant: Were they all the same person? Are some special events happening there?

Client: No, it seems that there were two or three involved, but I think that it would be useful for the rest of the department to be reminded of it.

Consultant: Well, I am certainly willing to do such a workshop. Let me ask another question. What would you like to have as the outcome of the workshop?

Client: Well, most immediately, I would like to have the complaints stop. The focus seems to be the answering of the telephones. I would like people to respond to the phones within three rings and answer them in a friendly manner.

Consultant: Let me do this. I will take this discussion and summarize it. Then I will send you a proposal to which you can respond that will contain a set of objectives for the workshop, possible agenda, and time frames. You can then get back to me and let me know if that is in the ball park. How does that sound?

Client: Sounds good to me.

Consultant: Okay. I will have this to you by Friday of this week.

Summary

This chapter has been about establishing an effective relationship between the internal consultant and the client. Our belief is that the relationship is ultimately the key to the productive consultation. If the relationship has been established in

Establishing an Effective Client Relationship 97

confusion and chaos, the outcome will probably not be successful. The lesson is that we need to be intentional in establishing a relationship that has potential for success.

This chapter has presented many ideas and thoughts on the topic of contracting. For us, good contracting is good consulting.

We encourage you to take the questions we have raised and to adapt them to your setting. You may want to make shortened versions of the contracting questionnaires in Exhibits 2 and 3. What is important is that you take the concept of contracting seriously in a way that is useful for you in your setting.

Remember that contracting is simply defining tasks and relationships so that the project can be accomplished. It is a tool that will allow you to more effectively use your most valuable resource — time.

Consultation Skills for Health Care Professionals

Exhibit 3. Contracting Skills Checklist.

The following is a listing of skills needed for internal consulting. For each skill, rate yourself as:

(+) — You are well skilled and competent in this skill.
(0) — You are okay in this skill.
(−) — You feel yourself lacking in this skill.

General Consultation Skills
___ 1. Ability to listen to others
___ 2. Ability to ask direct probing questions
___ 3. Ability to listen to self and be aware of own feelings
___ 4. Ability to understand organization
___ 5. Ability to get industry-specific information
___ 6. Ability to think before reacting
___ 7. Ability to be comfortable with education and skill background
___ 8. Ability to understand why in a helping profession
___ 9. Ability to separate personal from professional issues
___ 10. Ability to build an atmosphere of trust and openness
___ 11. Ability not to be needed
___ 12. Ability to say no
___ 13. Ability to let go
___ 14. Ability to take risks
___ 15. Ability to ask for help
___ 16. Ability to be flexible

Precontracting and Contracting
___ 17. Ability to negotiate, i.e., manage differences between you and others
___ 18. Ability to close a contract, i.e., reach agreements
___ 19. Ability to manage conflict and anger addressed at you
___ 20. Ability to manage conflict and anger addressed at someone else
___ 21. Ability to offer suggestions in an appropriate way
___ 22. Ability to draw out others, i.e., create a safe environment for them to share their ideas
___ 23. Ability to accept the client's definition of the problem and start from there
___ 24. Ability to help the client solve his or her own problems
___ 25. Ability to be honest to the client about what you can realistically deliver
___ 26. Ability to set realistic goals for the client and yourself
___ 27. Ability to help the client clarify the problem
___ 28. Ability to cost out projects in terms of resource consumptions
___ 29. Ability to think through the problem with the client in a logical sequence
___ 30. Ability to offer your own ideas freely
___ 31. Ability to provide the client with feedback in such a manner that it is most often heard and understood
___ 32. Ability to work with others whom you do not necessarily like or appreciate
___ 33. Ability to be flexible in your consulting style to meet the client's needs

5

Collecting and Analyzing Information

Now that you have entered into a contract and begun forming a relationship with the client, you are ready to start data collection and data analysis.

This chapter explores the various methods that can be used for data collection and techniques for data analysis. Our goal is to provide you with hands-on tools for both the collection and analysis of data, that is, for making sense of them. Without good data, the consult becomes meaningless. As our friends in the computer world say, "Garbage in, garbage out" (Gigo).

Earlier we said that most of the time the client does not articulate the actual problem but rather presents symptoms of the problem. Often when inadequate data are collected, symptoms of the actual problem get resolved—but guess what? The problem does not go away, and sometimes it even gets worse. Other times when inadequate data are collected, the "wrong" problem is solved. The end result is that much time, energy, and money on the part of the client and consultant have been wasted. Therefore, our job as internal consultant is to collect the necessary data needed to facilitate resolving the correct problem.

We have seen that the internal consultant wears many different "hats" in his or her role. Chapter Two discussed many of these roles—director, counselor, facilitator, and delegator. Now we want to add another hat—that of the detective. Much of the work of the internal consultant is detective work. What is really going on? How do we make sense of it? Imagine that you are a detective, and your job is to uncover clues and leads that will help you solve a major crime (problem). Imagine you are Jessica Fletcher (from "Murder She Wrote"), Agatha Christie (the famous mystery writer), or Sherlock Holmes, the most famous of all. Your role is to piece together the solution to the puzzle of the "crime." In the internal consulting analogy your role is to figure out the puzzle of what the problem is that the client needs resolved.

We have good problem-solving models in medicine. A patient might have presenting symptoms of increased appetite, increased urination, and fatigue. If the treating physician decided to act on the symptoms without gathering further data, he would discuss with the patient the importance of a well-balanced meal, drinking less fluids, and getting at least eight hours of sleep each night. Suppose the same patient decides to get a second opinion and goes to see another physician. This physician puts on her "detective" hat and performs a complete medical work-up, that is, gathering of family health history, X rays, blood work, urine tests, patient's medical history, weight variations in the past year, and so on. The end diagnosis, the problem that needs to be treated, is diabetes. In this case if the wrong problems were solved as a result of inadequate data collection, it would result in the patient's death.

Data collection and analysis are an integral part of the daily life of health care professionals: internal consultants, physicians, nurses, laboratory technicians, pharmacists, and psychosocial medicine practitioners. Their treatment modalities are very much based on the information and data that they collect. The result could be waste of resources and time or, in the extreme, life or death.

Other health care professionals (internal consultants) include staff in education, data processing, business office, marketing, development, public relations, environmental services, and materials management, who also base their activities on data or information that they collect. The results directly impact the viability of the department(s), which directly impact the entire organization.

Collecting and Analyzing Information 101

The next section will deal with methods of data collection, and the final section of this chapter will deal with data analysis. One note: clearly, it would be impossible for us to make you an expert in these topics in one chapter. Entire books have been written about them. However, we can give you hints and overviews. For those of you who want to learn more, use this as a stepping-stone to other books and resources. The next few sections are fairly detailed. Readers experienced in data collection and analysis may choose to scan these quickly. However, the detail may prove useful to less experienced readers.

Data Collection Methods

The first question is: How do we go about collecting data? However, this question should be asked only after you have decided what information is needed and who has that information. When you know what you want and from whom you want it, the next step is the selection of the best method of collection. The five standard ways of collecting data are:

1. *Questionnaires.* We see them everyday. When the cafeteria wants to know about its food, it sends out a questionnaire. When we want to know what the employees think, we send out an employee survey.

2. *Interviews.* A second major way to get or give information is through the interview, for example, in job interviews and exit interviews. Interviews can be formal or informal depending on the purpose and nature of the project on which you are working.

3. *Observation.* A third way to get information is through observation. Simply observe what is going on. Observation is an excellent way to get at the nuts and bolts of a situation. It allows you to find out firsthand what is happening in a particular situation.

4. *Reports.* This method simply uses what has already been done, for example, financial reports, incident reports, quality assurance reports, and so on. Every health care organization has a multitude of material that is already collected.

5. *Group interviews.* Group interviews are a special case of

the interview. The one method we will discuss is the sensing interview.

We believe that the best data collection involves two or more of the above methods. This is called triangulation. If more than one method gives the same information, the data are probably accurate.

The next few sections review the five data collection methods in some detail, outlining pluses and minuses of each along with some helpful hands-on suggestions.

Method 1: The Questionnaire

The questionnaire is probably the most famous data collection method. It is a quick way to get data from a wide variety of people. The advantages of questionnaires are many.

Questionnaire Pluses. The following are some questionnaire advantages.

1. *The ability to gather information from large numbers of people is a major questionnaire advantage.* When you find yourself needing to collect information from an entire department or from several departments, a questionnaire would be the method of choice. The beauty of the questionnaire is its portability.

2. *Questionnaires offer flexibility in that they can be distributed individually or to a group.* This means that they can readily be used with individuals or groups.

3. *Questionnaires can be applied to many populations and focus on a wide range of topics.* This makes them very versatile.

4. *Questionnaires provide the opportunity to ask open-ended as well as closed-ended questions.*

5. *Usually there is less risk taking on the part of the individual completing the questionnaire.* Names are generally not necessary, and confidentiality can be ensured. With sensitive material, this method tends to foster more open and candid responses, for example, when you are asking employees their opinion of their boss.

6. *Questionnaires can be more cost-effective in terms of time and*

Collecting and Analyzing Information

money. Once the questionnaire is developed, it is readily distributed to multiple audiences.

Questionnaire Minuses. A few disadvantages include the following.

1. *Preparing a questionnaire is often very time-consuming.* Once the questionnaire is prepared, basic reliability and validity testing is needed. Validity testing determines if you really are collecting what you think you are collecting. Reliability testing determines whether you will get consistent results with repeated measures.

2. *The return rate for mailed-out questionnaires is usually low, about 30 percent.* The key with mailed questionnaires is to "hook" the respondent. The more intriguing the respondent finds the questionnaire, the better the return rates will be. Often incentives—for example, money, coupons to a restaurant, pens, and so on—encourage participants to complete or return questionnaires.

3. *The individual receiving the mailed questionnaire does not have much opportunity to ask questions or discuss the issues.* This may lead recipients to misunderstand or misinterpret the questions or instructions. The result is poor data.

4. *Without using a true random questionnaire, results are less generalizable to the entire population (department, organization) being studied.* What we try to establish with random selection is for everyone in the population that we are studying to have an equal chance of being included, thus taking care of participant variances that may influence the findings. A simple way to randomly select participants is to put everyone's name in a hat and select by pulling out names until you get the desired number of participants.

5. *Information collected tends to be superficial.* While information may be in depth with well-designed questionnaires, questionnaires usually do not provide respondents with the option of asking questions for clarification.

6. *The information may be skewed because only certain types of people may return the questionnaire.* Typically, if you are asking questions about which some respondents have strong feelings,

those with the strong feelings (either positive or negative) will respond.

Questionnaire Hints. Here are some hints in the construction of questionnaires that we have found useful (Dunham and Smith, 1979):

1. *Take time to think about what information you want from the questionnaire.* Write down the information you want to collect. Try not to collect more information than you actually need. If you do not have a clear purpose in collecting information, then a rule of thumb is not to collect it.

2. *Based on the information you want, make your selection of the format for the questionnaire.* You may want to group the questions into sections within the questionnaire, for example, a demographic section with questions such as age, occupation, education level, and so on. Other sections might include data of what has happened in the past, and yet another section might focus on current issues.

3. *Take time to make your questions short and concise.* Long, garbled questions with two or three ideas tend to confuse the respondent. The standard types of questions are open ended and closed ended.

An *open-ended question* is one that allows the respondent to answer in his or her own words. An example is this: "What suggestions do you have for reducing turnover in this department?" Open-ended questions are most useful when you want to get people's feelings and thoughts about a topic and you are not sure how they will respond. Typically, the open-ended question is most useful when you do not know the categories in which people will respond. A major advantage is that open-ended questions do not force people into a certain kind of response but rather allow the respondent to say what he or she wants.

The disadvantage of the open-ended question is that you get lots of information that you really do not need. You may have difficulty pulling out the relevant facts.

There are several types of *closed-ended questions. Multiple-choice questions* are questions where several choices are shown, and the respondent simply indicates which responses are the

Collecting and Analyzing Information

most appropriate. The respondent may respond to one or a number of the choices. An example of a multiple-choice question is:

Which of the following is the most important cause of turnover in your department?

- low wages
- poor supervision
- benefit package

Multiple-choice questions are most useful when you know the key items for the response. For example, if we know the three key choices regarding turnover, multiple-choice questions make most sense. Multiple-choice questions are also quick to answer and easy to tabulate.

The major disadvantage is the opposite of the advantage. Multiple-choice questions force the respondent to respond to a certain set of items. If the respondent prefers a different item, there is no place to indicate it.

A *rating scale* allows the respondent to select a response according to a variant of ratings. For example:

How do you rate the current productivity system at the hospital?

5 = Excellent
4 = Good
3 = Fair
2 = Poor
1 = No comment

Rating scales can be effective in quickly gathering and analyzing data. Rating allows you to quantify the response in terms of importance instead of simple agreement or disagreement.

The major disadvantage is that the items need to be very well thought out or the data become meaningless. Also, there is a tendency for individuals to respond in the middle range. At times it is useful to word the responses in such a way that the respondent is forced into a favorable or unfavorable response. One example is use of a four-point scale such as this one:

4	3	2	1
Very good	Good	Poor	Very poor

The key with all types of questions is to keep them as simple as possible and word them in a way that is neutral so that the respondent does not feel led to a particular answer.

Later we will discuss each of these and some of their pluses and minuses.

4. *Once you have selected the questions, review them to see that they get you the information needed.* One of the most common errors is asking questions that you do not really need to ask.

5. *Take time to sequence the questions logically.* Remember, logic here is defined by the person filling out the questionnaire, not by the questionnaire's designer. This means that you have to think about how that person will respond to your questions. If you have various themes with which you are working (for example, in an exit employment survey a progression through pre-employment interview experiences, overall organizational experiences, and so on), all are separate phases. Jumping back and forth between these worlds most likely will cause frustration and confusion.

6. *Put the most important question first and the least important last.* If the respondent does not complete the questionnaire, the most important questions will have been answered.

7. *Be sensitive to the questionnaire instructions.* There is a tendency to write instructions in such a way that they make sense to you rather than to the respondent. This includes specific information such as whether you want the respondents to "circle" a response, "fill in a blank," and so on. Be sure to give instructions on when the questionnaire is to be returned and to whom.

8. *If appropriate, develop a cover letter to explain the purpose of the questionnaire.* The cover letter should contain information on what the questionnaire is about, how respondents were selected, why their information is important, how the information will be

Collecting and Analyzing Information 107

used, and time frames. An important part of the cover letter will be a statement about confidentiality. Finally, thank the participants for their cooperation.

9. *Take time to think about the presentation of the questionnaire.* How does it look? Is it neat? Attractive? If it looks like garbage, it probably will end up in the garbage.

Once you have done all this, step back from the questionnaire and imagine that you are seeing it for the first time. How would you respond if you were to get it in the mail? Would you complete it? A good idea is to "pilot test" the questionnaire by asking a few people to complete it and then discussing any difficulty or confusion they experienced.

Method 2: The Interview

One of the most valuable tools for data collection is the interview. We do interviews with one another all the time. "Do you want to go for coffee?" "To which movie would you like to go?" "What do you think is the most important task to be done in this department?"

The interview allows you to pursue the respondent's responses and to watch the verbal and nonverbal responses. You participate in the face-to-face interaction with the other person.

There are two major varieties of interviews. The first is the *structured interview*. In the structured interview, the questions are predetermined, and the interview proceeds like clockwork. In structured interviews, you know exactly the questions you want to ask and why. In the *unstructured interview*, you simply have a discussion with the respondent about her or his thoughts and views of the issue or problem. The discussion goes wherever it needs to go with no predetermined plan.

Interview Pluses. The major plus of the interview is that you can follow the client's lead. If the client wants to provide you with certain information, you can follow that lead. You can probe when the client hints that there may be more information, for example, with a statement such as "There is more than one reason why employees are dissatisfied with the new computer system." A probing question would be "What do you see as other reasons for the dissatisfaction with the system?" Unlike with the questionnaire, which does not reveal what the client is thinking, here you can find out what the client is thinking.

Another advantage is that of the interview relationship. In an interview the respondent is dealing with a real person instead of a cold piece of paper. That means the respondent can ask questions of clarification and that the interviewer can assess the nonverbal communication.

Interview Minuses. The minus of the interview is that the relationship can influence the interview outcomes. A dynamic interviewer can influence the interviewee by saying things such as "Did you really mean to say that...?" Also, the interview process is costly in terms of time and resources, and the interviewer needs a certain level of skills. Finally, the outcomes of the interview may be difficult to quantify and group.

Interviewing Hints. Here are some hints for the interview.

1. *Provide the respondent with pertinent information.* This includes the reasons for the interview, how the information will be used, how the respondent was selected to be interviewed, what your role in the interview is, and the time commitments involved.

2. *Make use of the first few minutes to build a relationship with the respondent.* Remember, the relationship quality of the interview is important. Take time to put the respondent at ease.

3. *Prepare for the interview.* Know what you want to get from it and the process through which you plan to go. Think about the room and how it needs to be arranged so that there is privacy for the interview.

4. *Think about how you want to keep track of the data from the interview.* Will you take notes during it? Will you tape it? Will you wait until the conclusion of the interview and then write down your notes?

Taking notes during the interview is the method that we use most frequently. It can be done in a nonobtrusive way so that the respondent does not become overly involved in watching you take notes. Jotting down main points or themes instead of

Collecting and Analyzing Information 109

every word the person says is best. The major disadvantage of taking notes is that the respondent may pick up clues as to what you want to hear by noticing when you write things down.

Taping during a session is another option. Taping allows you to attend to the interview and not worry about getting everything down on paper. It is important that the interviewee be aware that the tape is recording. Frequently, the interviewee's uneasiness with a tape will wear off in the first few minutes. The main advantage of taping is that you can come back to the tape and hear the words actually spoken. Our experience is that each time we listen to a tape, we hear some new data. The minus with the tape is that the interviewee may be uneasy about being recorded. (Who knows where they may hear it next?) Also, the interviewer may never get around to listening to the tape. Most of us do not have the time to listen to a tape over and over.

Taking notes after the meeting is another way to record interview data. The major advantage is that this method is very unobtrusive. It does not interfere with the session. The major problem is that the interviewer's memory is selective. He or she listens to and remembers only certain parts of the discussion.

5. *Be sensitive to nonverbal behaviors of the interviewee.* Remember that the major advantage of the interview is that it is face to face, so you can gather more information. The nonverbal behavior of the interviewee will provide you with significant data.

Sample Interview. The following is an example of an interview that we used when assessing management development needs with the ancillary departments.

Consultant: Thank you for taking time to meet with me. As you know, we are developing our management training program for next year, and we are asking directors what they see as the training needs of the management team. We will take the information that we gather from this and other interviews and use it in program development. As I mentioned on the phone, this should take only twenty minutes. Do you have any questions before we get started?

Client: Will my comments be attributed to me, or will they be confidential?

Consultant: Good question. No, your comments will not be attributed to you. We will make a summation of the comments, and your specific comments will not be identified with you.

When you think about the management team, what are the three top management development needs that you see?

Client: Are you asking for my needs or what I see with others?

Consultant: Both. What do you see as your needs and others' needs?

Client: Well, lots of my colleagues definitely need more skills in managing conflicts. They seem to be always fighting it out.

Consultant: Would you give me an example of one of the fights? What is going on? . . .

(Here the consultant begins to explore and probe the response. The goal is to get more information so that the need can be more accurately assessed. The consultant continues to explore until there is an understanding of the need.)

Consultant: So, it sounds like the issue is that some directors do not understand the role of other directors, and that is leading to conflicts. Is that an accurate statement?

Client: Right. We need some training in how we get clear role clarification.

(The process continues through the consultant's questions. The consultant is now ready to bring the discussion to a close.)

Consultant: One last question. Is there a question I have not asked you that you would have liked me to ask or something else that you would like to say about the topic?

Client: Only this. I think we need more sessions where the

Collecting and Analyzing Information 111

Consultant:
directors get together in an informal way and just get to know each other. We need more informal times together.

Thank you. I will be sure to mention that in my report. Again, I expect that I will be finished with the interviews in the next week. Then I will take that material and summarize it for the administrative team by early next month. You will receive a copy of that final report then.

Method 3: Observation

Perhaps the most common form of information gathering is direct observation. Think about that for a moment. For example, you are walking down the hall, and you see a piece of paper on the floor and pick it up. You had an observation and an action. Maybe you know that there are waiting problems in the outpatient area, so you structure a series of observations to see if you can detect what the problem is.

Observations are of two types. The first type is *random observation*, such as walking down the hall, seeing something, and responding to it. You had not planned an observation. You saw and reacted. Management by walking around is an example of random observation. The manager simply walks around the building and sees what is there.

The second type is *structured observation*. In the structured observation you plan in advance what it is for which you are looking and then proceed to make your observations. The observations are structured and formal.

Observation Pluses. The advantages of observation are:

1. *Observations collect data in real-life situations.* You are making observations of actual behavior, not speculating about the behavior. This makes observations very real.

2. *Observations allow the consultant an accurate, objective gathering of data.* With structured formal observations you simply follow your observation plan, for example, observing every tenth person you encounter.

3. *Observation does not impact the participants' work flow.* Observation is relatively unobtrusive—that is, it usually does not interfere with the work flow. Unlike questionnaires or interviews, which interrupt the individual, observations allow you to simply watch.

4. *Observations may be very simple to implement.* Again, observations can be as simple as walking out of your office and down the hall.

Observation Minuses. Disadvantages of the observation data collection method are:

1. *Individuals being observed often tend to act "differently."* Think about the last time you had someone watching you do your work. How did you respond to the fact that you were being watched? Remember Santa's warning—he is watching to see if you have been naughty or nice. Now, that changes behavior!

This change of behavior because of observation is known as the Hawthorne effect. It is essentially the concept that behavior is altered as long as the observation continues and then reverts to the previous behavior. The key learning is that simple observation can change behavior.

2. *Structured observation can be costly in terms of time and money.* Well-structured observations take time and energy. They do not happen overnight. First, you have to determine what is to be observed and by whom. Second, you have to develop the process for the observation, that is, when it will happen and how. All of this can consume resources.

3. *Often more than one observation of a situation is necessary.* Repeated observations of a situation may be necessary to ensure accuracy.

4. *Observer subjectivity impacts the observations.* The observer brings something to the observation, and that can contaminate the objectivity of the observations. The observer may see what he or she wants to see.

Observation Hints. Observation can be most useful, and it can be an exciting data collection tool. We often use observation when a client approaches us and requests assistance in finding

Collecting and Analyzing Information

the cause of a particular problem. The problem is clear. The consequences of the problem are clear. However, the etiology is unknown. Our example is one in which we were asked to analyze lengthy patient waiting times in the outpatient areas. That was the problem, but what was causing it? We did some observation of patients from the time of arrival until they walked out the door. We found not one cause for delays but many.

Some of the suggestions that we have for observations include:

1. *As with any data collection method, take time to plan the observations.* Know your purpose and how the observation can gather the data. It is wise to repeat the observation a few times to ensure that you are getting an accurate picture. There may be unusual circumstances or chance events that do not reflect normal occurrence.

2. *Establish the observation categories.* For structured observations, you need to identify what it is that you are observing. If you think about the work setting, there are hundreds of events and interactions every day — know which ones are important for you.

3. *After establishing the categories, develop the recording sheets for the data.* The sheets should provide you with a consistent method of observing and documenting the events.

4. *Establish your observation time frames.* Decide when and whom will you observe. Observing work in the outpatient clinic on a Monday at 8:00 A.M. will be quite different than observing work on Friday at 4:00 P.M. You need to know the work flow and how that impacts observations.

5. *Let the persons being observed know what is going on.* They need to know the purpose of the observations and what is happening with the data. Like with other methods, participants need to be informed.

On one project in a non–health care setting we were part of an eight-person observation team that turned up at the start of the workday unannounced. There were paranoia and hostility from the work force toward us, and rightfully so. We had appeared on their work scene unexpectedly.

Sample Observation. One example of observation is as meeting observer. The department director asked us to observe the meeting to provide her with hints on how the meeting might be run more effectively.

We established a checklist of items to be observed during the meeting. This included such items as:

- Participants are clear on the purpose of the meeting.
- Participants are clear on their role in the meeting.
- Participants are welcomed to the meeting, and an agenda is handed out with meeting events.
- The leader kept to the time frames of the meeting.
- The leader used flip charts to track the progress of the meeting.
- The leader demonstrated active listening skills.
- Actions attached to discussion items were recorded.
- Conflict was handled effectively.

The list was developed into a set of behaviors, and each time one of the behaviors appeared in the meeting, the observer made a note of it. At the end of the meeting the observer provided feedback on the meeting to the group.

Method 4: Reports and Records

So far, we have talked about methods of gathering data that impact the client group. Either we ask them questions or we watch what they do. Their work life is being intruded on.

Now we come to the one method of data collection that is unobtrusive. This is the use of existing records and reports. Think of the hospital setting and reports. Probably no organization keeps track of more records and reports than a hospital. Examples include performance reviews, quality assurance reports, risk management reports, incident reports, financial reports, end of the year reports, patient records, employee statistics, employee surveys, and exit interviews.

The list can go on and on. The point is that in all health care organizations much information is collected. For some

Collecting and Analyzing Information

types of consultations this information can be drawn on. A good example for us is a turnover study, which draws heavily on the exit interviews and other human resource information.

Some of the questions that you need to ask are:

1. What records and reports are currently being kept by the organization?
2. Do the current records contain information that is valuable to us on this project?
3. Will we have access to the information? Some records may not be opened to us due to their confidential nature.

It is important to know what is currently being collected and to be alert to how that might be useful to you.

Report and Record Pluses. There are a number of pluses with reports. First, their use is unobtrusive. You do not have to interfere in the life of the work group to get the data. Second, expense in accessing the information may be minimal. For example, from the exit reports you may get the same data that you would get from hours of interviewing. Third, reports can provide both quantitative and qualitative data.

Report and Record Minuses. The biggest plus, as we mentioned, is the amount of data already kept. This means that you do not have to reinvent the wheel. The minus is that while all those data are around, they may not be useful for you and this project. They may not be the kind of data you need. Second, the data may be old and not reflect the current situation. You may have a number of incident reports on something that once was a problem but has been corrected, but the historical record will still show a problem. Last, the conclusions may not easily be derived from the reports. You may be in a situation of comparing apples and oranges.

Report and Record Hints. There are some guidelines to use with reports and records. First, be clear about your data needs before you go after the reports. Know your purpose and what you are about. Second, develop a list of the current reports that might contain the data you are after. Third, have the necessary organizational backing to access the records. Fourth, be sensitive to the limitations of the reports. Be aware of the shortcomings.

Sample Reports and Records. A good example is our experience using reports and records in a turnover study. First we identified the records that might be useful. Exit interviews were one set of reports. The exit interviews contained the necessary information for us to form general conclusions regarding the reasons for the turnover. The second set of data was employee records. We were able to get basic employee information regarding supervisors, pay ranges, dates of hire, absenteeism, performance, and so on. Third, we looked outside our organization to the Bureau of Labor Statistics to get information on national trends.

Having developed a plan for action, our next step was to take that plan and get it sanctioned by the client and other key individuals such as human resources personnel.

Method 5: The Sensing Group

The sensing group (Jones, 1973, pp. 213–224) is a special type of group meeting held for the specific purpose of addressing a problem. Essentially, a sensing group is a group formulated to obtain viewpoints, suggestions, and wisdoms on a particular issue. For example, a sensing group may be formed around the issue of employee retention with the purpose of exploring ways that the organization can work with retention issues.

Essentially, a sensing interview is a group interview for the purpose of generating data to help determine what needs to be done.

Sensing Group Pluses. The advantages of the sensing interview are many.

1. *The consultant has the opportunity to verify his or her understanding of what the respondents are saying.* The responses can be

Collecting and Analyzing Information

expanded by soliciting examples from the person being interviewed. Also, since this is a group interview, others are there to validate or disagree with the discussion.

2. *The data from sensing interviews support and supplement data from other sources such as observation and survey techniques.* If the same phenomena emerge from several data-gathering techniques, the data become supportive of each other (Lawrence and Lorsch, 1969, p. 50). This is true of many methods. Typically, we like to use a questionnaire to prime the group and then have a group discussion. We will discuss this important point later.

3. *The act of interviewing members of the client system provides an opportunity for personal contact between the consultant and members of the client system.* This helps to reinforce the importance of the individuals in the client system.

4. *A climate of trust and openness can be established.* Again, the value of a group is that once there is a climate of openness, the group members may go into significant detail. This can readily help the consultant understand what is going on.

Sensing Group Minuses. It is equally important to be aware of the disadvantages of the sensing interview. Some of these include:

1. *Sensing interviews are time-consuming for the consultant and interviewees.* It can take a good deal of time to schedule the meetings and get everyone there.

2. *Often the data gathered from sensing interviews are not directly comparable to those gathered by other methods.* The data can be very subjective and need significant analysis.

3. *Data generated in interviews are not easily standardized or summarized.* This is an important point we will address later. Numbers are easy to summarize; a group's view on why the department is not working is not.

4. *Being interviewed may constitute a potential threat for the respondents.* The person being interviewed may be doing so involuntarily or reluctantly. There may also be people in the group who impact what will or will not be said.

5. *Groupthink—the phenomenon of the group members' all say-

ing the same thing—may be present. The result is that the data will be only partially useful.

Hints on Running Sensing Groups. A number of issues need to be thought through as the facilitator prepares for, engages in, and analyzes data from sensing interviews. Here are some of the keys to keep in mind.

1. *Preparing oneself.* The facilitator needs to be well prepared for the group. He or she needs to know what is wanted from the group and how those data will be used. This is critical.

2. *Preparing the interview.* The facilitator needs to have thought out the interview. He or she needs to know what questions to ask and in what sequence.

3. *Opening the interview.* Since the first few minutes are so important, they need special attention from the facilitator. Normally, the facilitator will begin with an objective of "breaking the ice" and warming up the group, perhaps with a story or a two-to-three-minute exercise. In addition, the facilitator needs to talk about the purpose of the group, who is there, and how the data will be used.

4. *Working on data gathering.* This is the section of the sensing interview where the information is actually collected, for example, through a survey, small group work, or the like.

5. *Closing the interview.* This is a time of group closure. It frequently is a very rich time because it is when the last ideas from the group can emerge.

6. *Analyzing the data.* A time-consuming part of the sensing interview is the data analysis, which is done by going back through all the data and making sense of them. (We will go into more detail with this in the next section.)

7. *Publishing the analysis.* This is the presentation of the data. This is a time for the consultant to reveal findings and recommendations.

There are some other points that we find important in working with sensing groups. First, the environment needs to be open and honest. The limits of confidentiality need to be explained carefully to ensure candidness. The usual approach is to establish that the data will be published anonymously. For exam-

Collecting and Analyzing Information 119

ple, instead of saying, "Paul, an evening staff computer analyst, is having problems communicating with Marguerite, the evening supervisor," the report might say, "A theme of ineffective communication flow between supervisors and employees came out in the group."

Second, the room should be comfortable. Attention needs to be paid to the physical meeting room area.

Third, interruptions should be limited. Do not allow beepers in the room.

Fourth, remember that participants may not be present on their own accord. They may have been sent. Therefore, there might be some resistance in the group. If resistance exists, it needs to be identified, discussed, and worked through before continuing with the interview. The consultant can watch for verbal and nonverbal clues that communicate resistance. We find that when we encounter significant resistance, it is important to mention it (for example, "Elizabeth, it appears that you are angry. Is that true?"). If the observation is confirmed, we try probing into reasons. Often it is a case of the employee's having incomplete information about the process or having strong feelings about this particular issue. In any case, identify such feelings, check with the interviewee, resolve, and move into the interview.

Fifth, it may be useful to begin the interview with questions that are anticipated to result in relatively little activity or emotion and to move toward more sensitive areas later in the interview, when a higher level of rapport has probably been achieved. The sequence of questions varies from situation to situation, and the model and sample questions in the sample sensing group below are designed to help explore and collect data for determining what needs to be done.

Sample Sensing Group. The following is a sample sensing group called together to develop ideas on health care futures. This group was initiated by the nursing department as part of the development of its five-year plan. The meeting was carefully planned to have refreshments on hand. The room was arranged in a manner that invited discussion. A round table was used so that all participants could see each other. The opening of the meeting and the selection of members were very deliberate. We had decided to tape the sessions and then do a content analysis of the tapes.

Consultant: The purpose of this group is to brainstorm about the future of health care and what will be needed in the year 1995. You have been selected as the participants because each of you represents a specific discipline that is an important part of the health care team. The results of this group will be used by nursing administration to develop the five-year plan for nursing.

When we invited you to the session, you were told that we would be taping the session. The purpose of the tape is so that we can listen to the session and pick out the main themes that emerge. That allows us to attend to what you are saying here without trying to remember what is going on.

Do you have any questions?

Group: How long will this take?

Consultant: It will take about one and a half hours. I will make sure that you are out by that time.

The place we would like to start is with this question: What is the growing edge in your particular department today for you? What is it that your professional societies are seeing as important?

(This is the start-up question. The group will then go on for some time with responses. If we notice a person not responding, we invite that person to respond more. After the warm-up time, we move into questions designed to focus the future.)

The above are some basic methods for data collection. There are also many variations on these basic themes.

We believe strongly that it is usually important to use more than one data collection method so that you can triangulate the data. Instead of doing just a questionnaire, do some interviews as well. If the data from both methods point in the

Collecting and Analyzing Information 121

same direction, you know that you are on the right track. If they point in different directions, you know you have more work to do. The important point is to use the multiple methods whenever possible.

Data Analysis

Now that you have collected mounds of data (many of us collect more than we need!), the key question to be asked is: What do I do with the data? How can I make sense of them? How can I take all the material from the questionnaire and interviews and whatever other methods that I utilized and make sense of those data? Or, more importantly, how do I let those data speak and make sense to me?

The internal consultant takes the lead in determining the important facts to report. What are the issues that stand out and have lots of energy attached to them? What are the trends in the data? These are the issues that need to be discussed with the client. If you are thinking about reporting every tiny piece of information you obtained—*don't*. You will end up with a mess. Key issues may go unnoticed, and everything will seem cluttered. Remember, the collection of data requires discrimination. Like picking flowers, selecting flowers worth picking and arranging them into a bouquet are ultimately matters of personal taste.

Block (1981) depicts helpful guidelines for selecting what to highlight to the client. Highlighted items need to include:

1. What the client has control over changing, things that he or she can do something about.
2. Items that are important to the organization.
3. Commitment somewhere in the organization to work on the item.

There are two basic approaches to data analysis. The first has to do with qualitative data, that is, data that are written comments or from interviews. Qualitative data are the respondents' comments regarding the questions and may or may not be quantifiable. The question for the consultant is: How do I make these data useful?

The second set of data is data that are quantifiable such as multiple-choice questions and rating scales. These are data to which you can put numbers.

Qualitative Data Analysis. Qualitative data are generally the most difficult to manage. They generally contain the respondents' comments, and the comments may vary greatly. In response to a question such as: What is not working in this department? you might get a full range of comments.

Yet qualitative data are sometimes the most valuable data. Here is how we deal with this type of data.

First, develop a listing of each theme in the data. Simply walk through the comments and write every new comment on a master theme list. If you have considerable data, this can be a large task, but it is needed for the next step.

Second, once the master list has been developed, go back to the data and start over. This time, your task is to build a frequency table for each theme. As you read through the data, put a check by each theme the respondent has identified on the master theme list. In this relatively easy manner you can arrive at a summation of the qualitative data that contains the major themes and their frequency. Usually if there are major themes this method reveals them quickly. A typical table would be like the one in Table 1.

In this particular situation, the top two themes were "ineffective communication flow between day and evening staff" and "supervisors seldom available to answer questions and help solve problems." These two items received the most attention and energy from the group. They are the key issues indicating attention and resolution.

The other use that we have for qualitative data is to reinforce quantitative data. For example, instead of simply providing some statistics that fifteen respondents reported ineffective communication between the day and evening staff, we provide some written comments such as:

Collecting and Analyzing Information

Table 1. Sample Theme Table.

Major Theme List	Response Frequency
Ineffective communication flow between day and evening staff	15
Supervisors seldom available to answer questions and help solve problems	13
Increased number of staff call-ins in the last two months	7
Staff not having access to updated policies needed to do the job	5
Ineffective staff meetings	5
Twenty percent increase in secretarial overtime in the past two months	2

Note: There were twenty participants in the group.

- Ineffective communication was more of a problem between the nurses and the secretaries.
- The problem is increased during the weekend due to staff shortages.
- Inadequate unit orientation on communication flow is part of the cause of the problem. (We provide some written comments. Providing this type of data to the client has the most impact.)

One last comment. If you are computerized, an outliner program can speed this process up considerably. A good package is MaxThink (trademark name), an idea processor used for thinking and writing. It is an outstanding tool for use with qualitative data analysis. (For more information contact Max-Think, 44 Rincon Rd., Kensington, Calif. 94707.)

Quantitative Data Analysis. Quantitative data are utilized when numerical values of a measurable character can be obtained. This type of data is a perfect match for computer analysis. In fact, numerous computer programs now available make this type of data analysis much easier.

Why use statistics? Fitz-Gibbon and Morris (1979) suggest

three major reasons for putting data into some form of statistics. First, statistics provide a means of summarizing data. The use of percentages, for example, can help us understand hundreds of responses. Second, statistics provide a means of measuring how serious differences are. Statistics help us understand if results are a product of chance or are fairly intentional. Third, statistics allow us to identify relationships between sets of data. For example, we might want to compare one group of people who stay in a department with those who leave a department.

Our use of statistics is basic and falls into two categories. The first is *descriptive statistics*, which are used to describe and summarize data.

The mean (average), median, and standard deviation are the main descriptive statistics. They are used to indicate the average score and the variability of scores for the sample being studied. The advantage of descriptive statistics is that they enable the researcher to use one or two numbers (for example, a mean or standard deviation) to represent all the individual scores of subjects in the sample! The reduction of mass raw data to a few descriptive statistics greatly simplifies analysis. However, oversimplification of data can occur. When the researcher does not examine the raw data, she or he may overlook important patterns and phenomena revealed by individual scores.

Let us take a closer look at how the internal consultant can use descriptive statistics in analyzing data. Several months ago a nursing director approached us and requested that we work with her to help improve the department's weekly staff meeting. She wanted to get a handle on exactly what was causing the recent influx of negative comments from the staff about the meetings. There were nine staff each on the day shift and the evening shift. The director requested that we look at the two groups separately. We started by asking the two groups about their perception of the effectiveness of the staff meetings. A ten-point scale was used to indicate effectiveness, with 1 indicating ineffectiveness and 10 effectiveness. We calculated the mean (average) for both groups. This provided us with a nice snapshot of where the groups were with this particular issue, as shown in Table 2.

Collecting and Analyzing Information

Table 2. Sample Data: Day and Evening Shift Responses.

Day Shift Responses		Evening Shift Responses
	7	2
	2	4
	3	6
	6	7
	5	2
	4	3
	7	2
	2	2
	1	1
Sum	37	Sum 29
Mean	4.1 (37/9)	Mean 3.2 (29/9)

The day shift was the first group analyzed. The mean was calculated by adding together all of the responses from the staff members and then dividing the sum (in our case, 37) by the number of staff (in this case, 9). The mean response of the day shift was 4.1. Similar calculations were conducted for the evening shift, and the mean was 3.2.

The next calculation was the median. The median is the middle score in the distribution of scores. Fifty percent of the cases fall below the median, and 50 percent of the cases above the median. It represents a typical value. The median for the day shift was 5, and for the evening shift 2.

An important characteristic of the median is that it does not take into account the quantitative values of individual scores. The median is simply an index of average position in the distribution of numbers. The median is not sensitive to extreme values. It is useful when the distribution is skewed (weighted to one side) and one is interested in finding a typical value, such as in the following lists of numbers:

8 7 6 6 6 10 9 5 8   (median = 6)
8 7 6 6 6 10 9 5 800 (median = 6)

The mean is considered the best measure of central tendency, that is, the single numerical value that is used to describe the average of an entire sample of scores. Computing the mean is usually necessary before applying more of the advanced statistical tools such as standard deviation, analysis of variance, and so on. If we study several samples from the same population, the mean scores are likely to be in closer agreement than median scores.

The final descriptive statistic that we will review is the standard deviation. It measures the extent to which scores in a distribution on the average deviate from their mean. Like the mean, the standard deviation takes into consideration every score in the distribution. Like the mean, it provides a way of describing group scores on the basis of a single measure.

The mean and standard deviation, taken together, usually provide an excellent description of the nature of a group. One step in calculating the standard deviation is to subtract each score from the mean. The resulting deviation scores are then squared and entered into a formula to give the standard deviation. It is a popular measure of variability because it is stable (that is, standard deviations are usually similar when drawn from the same population).

The second category of statistics is *inferential statistics*. We use these when we need to infer and draw conclusions from as well as describe data. For example, assume the internal consultant is asked to find out the commitment level of the staff. She has two hundred randomly selected members of the nine hundred staff with whom to work. She finds that among the sample there is low staff commitment to the organization. With the assistance of inferential statistics, she can generalize the results to the nine hundred employees based on the results of the two hundred staff. That is the essence of inferential statistics.

We have chosen to close our discussion of statistics at this point. Readers who wish to explore the subject further should check Block (1981) and Fitz-Gibbon and Morris (1979).

Uses and Abuses of Statistics

Statistical methods are tools for rendering large amounts of data useful. Basic knowledge of statistical methods enables

Collecting and Analyzing Information

the consultant to take the information gathered and make it understandable and digestible. It allows the consultant to reduce, summarize, organize, evaluate, interpret, and communicate numerical information.

There are some pitfalls to keep in mind when working with statistical data. *First, be clear about the sources of the statistics.* A danger is to develop a very finely tuned statistical analysis based on a poorly developed questionnaire. In such a case, the statistics may look excellent but the foundation on which they are built is very weak.

Second, be conservative in your use. One of the beauties of computers is that they can generate detailed statistics. Their downside is that they allow us to drown the client with statistical output.

Third, with all types of reporting, present the data clearly. If the statistics are inconclusive, say so. If the data have conflicts in them, say so. Do not set aside some of the data because they do not support your view.

Fourth, use the data for the purpose for which they were intended.

Remember the basics. The intent of data analysis is to take a multitude of written and numeric comments and make sense of them, or, as we like to say, put them in a form that can speak clearly. Let the data talk to you so you can make decisions regarding them.

Exhibit 4 provides a checklist of the skills necessary for data collection and analysis.

Conclusion

This chapter has been about data collection and analysis. We present it humbly, because any one topic in this chapter is worth several books in and of itself. Data collection and analysis are the foundation for the rest of the consulting process, which depends on how well this step has been done. If it is done poorly, the rest of the process is at risk. It is like the diagnostic procedures of a physician—the treatment is only effective when there has been accurate diagnosis.

In this chapter we have identified the major methods for

Exhibit 4. Data Collection and Analysis Skills Checklist.

The following is a listing of skills needed for data collection and analysis. For each skill, rate yourself as

(+) — You are well skilled and competent in this skill.
(0) — You are OK in this skill.
(−) — You feel yourself lacking in this skill.

Data Collection and Analysis
___ 1. Ability to determine a plan of data collection, analysis, and presentation
___ 2. Ability to determine the data needed for a consultation
___ 3. Ability to obtain data needed for a consultation
___ 4. Ability to design questions that get the needed information for questionnaires and interviews
___ 5. Ability to use library resources in obtaining data
___ 6. Ability to use computers for data collection and analysis
___ 7. Ability to recognize and explore a broad range of ideas and practices
___ 8. Ability to store data in an easily retrievable manner
___ 9. Ability to take complex ideas and processes and present them as models so that the models capture the complex processes
___ 10. Ability to review collections of written comments and pull out the common themes
___ 11. Ability to use basic statistical processes to make sense of data
___ 12. Ability to integrate diverse sources of data
___ 13. Ability to take complex data and reduce them to common themes and make sense of them
___ 14. Ability to do cost-benefit analysis

---

data collection and have discussed advantages and disadvantages of each. Our goal is to leave you with sufficient information that you will be able to select the best method for your situation.

Finally, in this chapter, we have talked about "formal data collection." Remember, you are constantly in the process of receiving data from the client. During the interviews you are getting data not only in response to the questions but also from how the client is reacting to the questions, and at times those are the most important data. We say that all encounters with the client supply us with data. Our task is to make sense of them.

The next chapter begins to discuss the question: So I have done all this data collection and analysis. What now?

6

Presenting the Data

One of the most exciting phases in the consulting model is the communication of findings to the client. Your job as internal consultant is to present a clear, concise, objective snapshot of your data.

The purpose of this chapter is to give you suggestions in preparing the report and orchestrating the meeting. We will look at communicating findings one on one (consultant and client) as well as to a group.

The presentation of data may be to a group or to an individual. It may be written or verbal. We will provide examples of formal and informal types of feedback meetings.

An important purpose of the feedback meeting is to have the client react to the data that you have collected and analyzed. The presentation time is a final check on the data—do the data make sense to the client? Does the client think that some things were missed? What about the recommendations? Do they make sense to the client? This means that you need to be open to having the client disagree with all or part of your data.

One last comment by way of introduction. We have chosen to go into detail with the presentation process. The more experienced reader may want to skim the material and compare our suggestions with his or her own experience.

The Presentation Process

The presentation process is composed of three parts. The *first part is the preparation for the meeting.* This is a time of deciding what will be presented, how, and when. This is a time of thinking about types of visual aids that might be used to facilitate the presentation.

The *second part is the meeting itself*. Here we have questions about who will manage the meeting and how the material will get presented.

The *third part is the meeting follow-up*. It is important to have a follow-up to the meeting to summarize it.

Remember, the best collection of data with the best analysis will go nowhere if the data are poorly presented. Do not undermine the work of the previous steps by inadequate preparation at this time.

Premeeting Preparation

We have found the CPR + F model useful in preparing for the presentation meeting. We suggest that prior to the meeting the consultant think through the four main parts of the model:

- *Purpose.* Be clear on the purpose of the meeting. Do what you need to do to make sure the client group is also clear with the purpose of what will be happening.
- *Commitment.* Think about the participants' levels of commitment. What levels of commitment do you think the various key players are bringing to the meeting?
- *Roles.* Have the roles for the meeting been clearly defined? Do the parties to the meeting have an agreement about such things as who will run the meeting and what is expected of each of them as participants?
- *Feedback.* What will be the indicators that the meeting is staying on track? How will we determine if the meeting's outcomes have been met? The question is one of feedback: What will the feedback channels be?

The CPR + F model can be useful as we think through the general meeting design. Here are some specific guidelines that we have found important in preparing for the meeting:

Plan your strategy for the meeting. Take time to think through

Presenting the Data

what you want by way of outcomes. With what would you like to leave the meeting? For what outcomes are you looking? What do you want from the other participants? Do you want them to actively engage in discussion about the data you have collected? Do you want them to vote on the conclusions?

Take time to think about when during the day you would like to hold the meeting. Some people are more morning people; others come alive in the evening. We generally prefer to hold the meeting midmorning if possible. By then people have had time to get to work and get started but are not too far into the day to be worn out.

However, once again, let the purpose determine the time. You may need to hold the meeting off site. The good news is that this gets you away from the immediate demands at work. The realistic side of this is that you must have the meeting when everyone can attend.

Plan for the meeting setting. Think about the setting in which you will be. How do you want the room set up? What is the atmosphere that you want to create?

A private, spacious, comfortable room should be selected for the meeting. Remember—the setting can have a favorable impact on the meeting and its outcomes. Do not hold an important meeting in the back of the cafeteria unless that is your only option.

Assuming that we want the client group to interact with us, we try to make sure that the room is set up in a manner that invites interaction. For groups of people we recommend a circular table-and-chair or chair arrangement. This arrangement facilitates eye contact, promotes inclusion, and encourages participation.

Plan for agendas and advance material. For many meetings it is best to send out materials to the participants ahead of time so they have an opportunity to prepare for the meeting. Sometimes this is simply an agenda; at other times it is something much more extensive.

Keep faith with what was said during the contracting. If you said you would deliver the information to a certain group of people, make sure that you do. Do not leave out some people unless there has been an intentional change of the contract.

Go back to the contract and see who was listed as needing to be part of this time. This can be usually left to the discretion of the client. We suggest including the client department/group most impacted by the issues and those who are needed to help in the planning and resolution of the issues. On occasion we have suggested that the client's boss or other administrative personnel be included. This largely depends on the nature of the findings and its impact on other departments or the organization.

Think about your audience. What are their expectations of the meeting? What will be the best way to present your data to them? Will they want to see overheads? Will they want to discuss what has been presented, or will they have agendas of their own?

Keep the client in an active role in the meeting. We believe strongly that the client needs to be seen as the leader of the meeting. That may be accomplished by something as simple as having the client start the meeting and then turning it over to you. Your role is to work within the framework that the client sets and make the client look good.

Written materials require a good amount of preparation time. Here are some guidelines for written materials:

Keep any reports or written materials trim. Do not include every piece of information that you collect. Sort through and report information in common themes. Look for information with lots of energy attached to it, that is, information in which the client seemed most interested. Also, look for data that have departmental or organizational importance and about which the department or organization can reasonably do something. If you present a twenty-page report, probably nobody will read it. Twenty-page reports are sometimes necessary. However, our goal is an executive overview that is two or three pages long with appendixes.

Make it understandable. Avoid statistical jargon and reporting that few people are likely to understand. Present supporting data and use charts and graphs to present and summarize data. Make the data as visual as possible.

Report the data objectively. Do not use your influence to sway

Presenting the Data   133

decisions one way or the other. Your opportunity for input will come. One of the best ways to monitor our own biases is to make the client aware of them.

Structure the meeting so you will have adequate time for discussion. Filling an agenda so full that there is no time to discuss the findings can be a problem. Make sure there is time for discussion.

Review wording of the report to ensure that it is nonevaluative. In some settings you may want to be evaluative. However, your role is to present the data in a manner that provides "the facts and nothing but the facts." If you are going into the meeting with many biases, plan how to manage them in the meeting.

Determine which elements of the report are likely to generate client defensiveness. Know where and what the hot buttons might be. Do not avoid them, but plan to take time to think through what they might mean and how you might manage them.

We like to use the following structure in the report itself:

1. Overview of the problem(s)/issue(s). You may refer back to the original contract and identify what was discussed there.
2. Discuss the process that you used for data collection and analysis. If there is bias in the data, mention this, thus giving the reader full information so he or she can decide how to weight the data in the report.
3. Present the data actually collected. It is easy to get sidetracked and spend time on projecting and speculating about information that was not collected.
4. Present the implications and recommendations based on the data. In some settings this meeting may be to develop next steps or make recommendations. If this is the case, leave this section blank.

Plan for your audiovisual equipment requirements. How many times have you attended a presentation where you could not see what was being projected on the overhead or slide? This can be very distracting and frustrating. In such a case, instead of enhancing the group, the audiovisuals cause the group to struggle to understand. The key to presentation is to get your message across. If this does not happen, information can be lost.

Audiovisual needs depend on the preferences of the consultant and the types of materials planned for the meeting. We tend to use three major types of AVs:

1. *Overhead transparencies.* One of the advantages of using overheads is that you do not have to dim the room lights. You are able to maintain eye contact with the group while having the material well organized and presented. Another advantage is that you can add material to the AV as you present the material. You can write on the overhead to add items the group may bring up. Still another advantage is that you can use the overheads over and over. Another is that the overhead serves the function of focusing the group in one direction. Last, overheads are easy to use and inexpensive.

One disadvantage of the overhead is the group can get distracted if the overhead projector is noisy. Another disadvantage is that overheads can direct the discussion too much in one direction. Still another is that if the overheads are not put together well, they may be difficult to read.

2. *Slides.* Major advantages of slides are the color and the preplanning. When you walk in with slides, you communicate to the group that the agenda is laid out and things are written in permanent ink—and they are on your slides. The presentation is sequenced ahead of time. Also, slides can be used with small or large groups. Slides are reusable and are readily carried from one setting to another. In general, well-prepared slides communicate preparation and quality to the audience.

The major disadvantage of slides is that they do not allow for additions from a group. The sequence is set prior to the meeting. Also, the lights usually have to be dimmed and therefore contact with the audience can be lost while slides are being shown. Slides can also be costly to make. The major weakness is perhaps also a strength—slides can communicate to the group a sense of a finished product instead of a product that is evolving.

3. *Flip charts.* Flip charts have the advantage of evolving as the meeting evolves. They are most useful in keeping a record of what has happened in the discussion. In addition, flip charts can

Presenting the Data

be readily added to and deleted from. This communicates to a group that they are in the process of editing and creating the product. Flip charts can also be prepared ahead of time, allowing you to lay out what you want to say at the meeting. You can prepare flip charts with material prior to the meeting, and you can keep track of the meeting's progress on the flip charts. Flip charts are relatively inexpensive.

A disadvantage is that if you spell or write poorly, the audience may have trouble reading your flip chart. Flip charts are more difficult to carry around than a set of slides. (We know this from having lugged flip charts all over the country.) In addition, flip charts are not good for large audiences, because they have difficulty reading a flip chart.

Mostly we use flip charts and overhead transparencies. Two excellent resources for preparation of flip charts are Geoffrey Ball (1978) and Richard Brandt (1986). Whether you use overheads, slides, or flip charts, it is important to remember a few cardinal rules.

- Do not clutter the slide or overhead. Clutter tends to be very distracting, causing the audience to tune out. The rule of thumb is no more than six lines apiece. An example of the worst kind of overhead would be one that contains the complete income expense sheet for the organization and is out of focus.
- If you use graphs or charts, be sure that they can be adequately projected in order for them to be seen by everyone.
- Limit the number of slides or overheads used. A good rule of thumb is one every five minutes. Remember, you want to have time for discussion.
- Do not project a slide or transparency and then talk about another subject matter. The group will be confused looking at an overhead that has nothing to do with the discussion.
- Always have extra felt-tip markers, flip-chart paper, projector, and overhead light bulbs on hand. As the Boy Scouts say, be prepared.

Austin (1981, pp. 161–169) has developed a checklist to help in selecting AVs. Some of his questions are:

1. Would AVs enhance your offering?
2. Do you have access to the desired material?
3. Do you have the equipment necessary to use the AVs?
4. Are the AVs suitable for the desired purpose?
5. Have you planned how to derive maximum benefits from the audiovisuals?
6. Are you knowledgeable with using the AVs?

You can use the Austin list to help decide whether or not to use AVs.

Do not invite beepers to the meeting. Beepers and phone calls are natural and very important for the health care professional. However, they tend to create major disruptions in meetings and presentations. We strongly encourage group participants to have a colleague take the beeper during the meeting and hold calls as much as possible. This effort will do much to facilitate the meeting's flow and continuity.

Practice the presentation. Perhaps this sounds a bit regimented, but we recommend taking time to think through and walk through the presentation. Remember that the presentation is judged on the material and how it comes across. Take some time and practice a walk-through. What will you be saying when, and how does that match with any AVs that might be used? Practice in front of a mirror or get some people together and do a dry run with them. Here are some practicing guidelines:

- Present one point at a time and build to the larger picture.
- Use examples, analogies, and graphics to help get your points across.
- Avoid jargon and keep the language basic.
- Plan when you will involve the participants and how. Remember, a question like "Are there any questions?" might get blank stares, whereas a question like "What is the question you have in your mind?" will probably lead to more discussion.

Presenting the Data 137

Exhibit 5. Premeeting Planning Form.

The purpose for the meeting is:

For this meeting to be a success, the following things need to happen:

Has the agenda for the meeting been prepared? Yes ___ No ___
Has the purpose for the meeting been agreed to by the client and yourself? Yes ___ No ___
Have the participants in the meeting been informed of their role in the meeting, that is, what is expected of them? Yes ___ No ___
Does the agenda include time for discussion of items? Yes ___ No ___
Have the room location and arrangement been confirmed? Yes ___ No ___
Have the participants been informed regarding date, time, location, and agenda? Yes ___ No ___
Have participants been sent advance materials for preparation? Yes ___ No ___
Has the AV equipment been arranged for? Yes ___ No ___
Have you prepared for the meeting and identified potential hot spots in the agenda? Yes ___ No ___

- When you are in the discussion phase, avoid arguing with the participants. Remember, you do not have to defend the data. Do not become defensive.
- Think about your personal appearance and plan how that will be part of the environment you want to create.

Remember that you are not expected to have all the answers in your role as internal consultant. Your responsibility is to present the facts and facilitate the meeting, moving it along to the next phase of the consulting model, the action phase or the implementation.

The overall goals for the individual or group meeting are to deliver the data, facilitate the meeting, and have the client(s) take responsibility for the situation and planning the next steps. A premeeting planning form is provided in Exhibit 5.

Once the preparation for the meeting has occurred, you will move into the second part of the presentation process, the meeting itself. This may take many forms. The two most common are the one-on-one meeting where you and the client meet alone together, or the presentation to a group of some type.

One-on-One Meeting with the Client

The one-on-one meeting with the client is the opportunity for the consultant to present the client with an overview of the data. A concise written report of the findings is suggested. The written report needs to include a listing of the key issues, positive and negative circumstances surrounding the issues, recommendations, and next steps. One-on-one meetings give the client an opportunity to react to the findings, which are sometimes good and sometimes not. If the client were to become angry and defensive in front of a group, it would have serious consequences for group participation in the meeting. A one-on-one meeting gives the client the opportunity to work through feelings and ask questions and the time to prepare for the group meeting. The one-on-one meeting should occur about two to three days prior to the group meeting.

The consultant and client now begin to prepare for the group meeting. Both are actively involved in planning the meeting agenda. It is important to establish criteria of success for the meeting (for example, what a successful meeting would look like, what would need to happen for it to be successful, and so on), in addition to the agenda.

Group Presentation Session

Table 3 shows a typical agenda that we might follow in the presentation meeting. The fourteen steps presented in Table 3 can be readily added to and subtracted from. They represent the general design for the feedback meeting. Some considerations that we feel important are:

1. *The client introduces the agenda and purpose of the meeting to the group.* It is important that the client take the lead role in reviewing her or his support of the process and the meeting, briefly recap what has happened up to this time, and pro-

Presenting the Data

Table 3. Sample Agenda for Presenting Data.

What	Who	Resources
Introduction		
1. Recap events of consulting contract that have occurred to present time.	Client	Flip chart; overhead; printed material
2. State support for consulting process and meeting.	Client	—
3. Create an open, safe, supportive, participative atmosphere.	Client	—
4. Present purpose for meeting and give overview of agenda. Discuss roles of consultant and client in meeting.	Client	Flip chart; overhead
Report		
5. Overview of key issues and problems.	Consultant	Flip chart; overhead; printed material
6. Present factors that are causing problem(s)/issue(s). These are factors that need to be stopped.	Consultant	Flip chart; overhead; printed material
7. Present factors that are not occurring but need to start. Break into short- and long-term goals.	Consultant	Flip chart; overhead; printed material
8. Present positive factors surrounding situation. These are factors that need to be continued.	Consultant	Flip chart; overhead; printed material
Feedback		
9. Feedback/reaction from group to report. Ask for levels of agreement.	Consultant, client	Group discussion
10. Ask group for additions to report.	Consultant, client	Group discussion; flip chart
Discussion		
11. Discuss benefits and nonbenefits of following through with action plan.	Consultant, client	Group discussion; flip chart
12. Check energy to assess group's willingness/desire to resolve problem	Consultant or client	Flip chart; use a ten-point scale to help quantify
13. Next steps: mapping out blueprint for action	Client	Group discussion; flip chart
14. Summary/conclusion; recap major issues and next steps.	Consultant	Flip chart

vide an overview of the contract and the "journey" that has been taken. The client should also set her or his expectations for the meeting. For example, those expectations might include:

An open, honest, and safe atmosphere
Participation invited from everyone
Freedom to ask questions and listen to others
Freedom to agree and disagree without consequence
Taking of a proactive rather than a reactive stance

Having the client introduce the agenda and purpose will serve to empower the client. The roles of the consultant and client in the meeting are discussed. The client is the leader; the consultant is the facilitator.

2. *The internal consultant presents the report.*
   A. Overview of the key issues. The internal consultant presents the factors that are causing the problem(s) based on the data collected. These are the factors that need to be addressed. The consultant also presents the factors that are not occurring but need to occur. These are best broken down into ones requiring either short-term or long-term planning. The positive factors surrounding the situation need to be presented as well—these are factors that need to continue.
   B. The consultant asks for reaction to the report. What were the "surprises"? What were the unexpected findings? The consultant asks for accuracy/agreement with the findings. What are things with which the group disagrees? What are things that need to be added?
   C. The consultant leads a discussion regarding the benefits of following through with the action plan. What are pitfalls of the action plan? What are some places where the plan may get stuck? What happens if we do nothing?
3. *The client assesses the group's energy level to move into the action phase to help resolve the problem.* This can be quickly and easily obtained using a ten-point scale. The purpose is to check on the group's investment in the process. The energy of the group is its fuel.

Presenting the Data

4. *The consultant, client, and group make plans for the next steps.* What needs to happen? Who needs to be involved? How will it happen? What will the time frame be? And so on.
5. *Summary/conclusion.* This is a brief (five-minute) recap of the major issues and an outline of the next steps.

Postsession Follow-Up

The feedback meeting is over. Now it is time to review the meeting. Here are a few questions you might ask:

1. What purposes/goals were set for the meeting? Were they met? If not, why not?
2. What was the outcome of the meeting? Did it meet the "success criteria" that you and the client established earlier when planning the meeting? How did this happen or not happen?
3. What were the things that you liked about the meeting? What were the learnings—the things that you did not like, the roadblocks? What would you change if you were to do the meeting again?
4. What was the reaction to the report? Surprise, agreement, disagreement, anger, apathy? How were these reactions introduced, received, and worked with in the meeting, by both the client and the group?
5. Was it an effective meeting? Was the open, trusting, participative climate established and perceived by the group? Was there resistance in the group? If so, how did this occur, and how was it resolved?
6. What were the nonverbal messages in the meeting? What did these represent? Did they facilitate or hinder the success of the meeting? How were they managed?
7. Were there a discussion of next steps and agreement to continue the consulting project? Does enough energy and enthusiasm exist to resolve the problems?
8. What were the key learnings from this meeting?

142   **Consultation Skills for Health Care Professionals**

Exhibit 6. Meeting Summary.

Was the purpose of the meeting accomplished? Yes ___ No ___
Were the desired outcomes achieved? Yes ___ No ___
If not, what outcomes were not achieved?

What action steps came out of the meeting, and who is to accomplish them by what time?

Action to Be Taken   *By Whom*   *By When*

Items that need to be carred over to a future agenda include:

Items   *Who Responsible*

The next step would be a discussion and sharing of your responses to the above questions with the client. A meeting summary form is provided in Exhibit 6.

Now you are almost ready to move into yet another phase of the consulting sequence: taking steps to act. Before moving into this phase, you should complete the presentation skills checklist in Exhibit 7.

Conclusion

This chapter has been about the presentation of the results of data collection and analysis. The important message is this: data do not necessarily sell themselves. Assume that you will need to sell the data. Remember, regardless of how effective you have been in the first few steps, if you do not present the data in a manner that the client will receive, the data will be lost.

Presenting the Data

Exhibit 7. Presentation Skills Checklist.

Internal Consulting Skills
The following is a listing of skills needed for internal consulting. For each skill, rate yourself as:
- (+) — You are well skilled and competent in this skill.
- (0) — You are okay in this skill.
- (−) — You feel yourself lacking in this skill.

Data Presentation
___ 1. Ability to project trends and potential futures
___ 2. Ability to put together written reports regarding data and analysis
___ 3. Ability to present data analysis using verbal communications skills
___ 4. Ability to manage questions placed to you
___ 5. Ability to select the appropriate AV materials for presentations
___ 6. Ability to work with groups and teams in presenting and discussing the data

7

Taking Action and Evaluating the Results

Learning, change, and action cannot take place without valid and reliable information. An organization relies on systematic data collection on which it then takes steps to act to accomplish its goal of improving departmental and organizational effectiveness.

The purpose of this chapter is to explore the consultant's and client's roles in the implementation phase and the evaluation phase. We will look more closely at the action step responsibilities and evaluation with a walk-through starting with the objectives, time line, resources required, use of written contracts, and follow-up letter of understanding.

We have used action planning as a common thread throughout the consulting project. Action planning was part of relationship building and contracting, data collection, and implementation. We now focus on action planning as a topic of its own.

The overall goal of action planning is to empower the client, not only in this phase of the project but throughout. The consultant facilitates and guides the client in using the feedback information as a stimulus for change. A bridging of the gap—that is, movement from the present state to the desired state—occurs.

Taking Action and Evaluating the Results

The Action Plan: Steps to Achievement

The first step is formulation of the objective. Once again, the contracting process and data analysis will be very informative in clarifying the objective. The client and consultant need to establish an action plan with the following parts:

1. an objective
2. tasks to complete
3. task start and end dates
4. identification of responsible person
5. resources needed
6. costs involved

We describe these in detail in the following sections. Again, the more experienced internal consultant may choose to flip through quickly; however, the detail may prove useful for the less experienced internal consultant.

The Objective. What does the client want to accomplish? What is the desired end state? Once this is established, the action process begins. Essentially, the action plan is the process designed to bridge the gap between current state and desired state. The objective is what sets the course of the action plan.

The objective should be written as an outcome measure, meaning that the objective is stated in terms of the future condition (for example, "When this project is complete, we will reduce turnover by 15 percent"). This is an outcome measure.

The action plan can have more than one objective. In some projects there will be several.

Tasks to Complete. Once the objective has been established, the next step is to list the tasks necessary to meet the objective. First list the tasks and then sequence and prioritize them. Some steps will need to occur before others, and some will be more vital than others. Know the priorities and importance of each.

Exhibit 8. Tasks to Be Done.

1. Inform the participants of the project	xx
2. Design questionnaire.	xxxxxxxx
3. Design cover letter to questionnaire.	xxxxxx
4. Send out questionnaire.	x
5. Begin analysis.	xxxxxx
6. Write final report.	x
	Day 1 2 3 4 5 6 7 8 9 10

Task Start and End Dates. It is useful to put a start date and an end date for each task. That allows you to build a calendar of activities. Later in this chapter we talk about the use of computerized project planners. There are some complex systems and some simple systems that can be most useful for this section.

On smaller projects the start and end dates may be the start and end dates of the project rather than of a specific task. The objective is to be able to have the project laid out along a time line.

A Gantt chart is one example of showing the tasks laid out along a time line. A Gantt chart simply lists the tasks that need to be accomplished with the time frame needed for each task, as shown in Exhibit 8.

Identification of Responsible Person. Who will be responsible for this particular task? Depending on the project's size, one person may have the total responsibility for the project, or responsibilities may be delegated. What is important is that a specific person be assigned to each task.

Resources Needed. Resources include both material and people. The human resources department deals with how many and what type of people will need to be involved in carrying out the project. In some settings this is a listing of the departments that need to be involved in the project or tasks.

Material resources are the items that will be needed to get the task done. Perhaps this is a computer and computer soft-

Taking Action and Evaluating the Results 147

ware, or maybe office supplies. It might be a room out of which an implementation team will work. These are the key resources needed for the project to be successful.

The consultant and client need to ask: Are the resources readily available in the organization? Or would it be better to have the implementation phase of the process done by an external consultant? Even though the consultant has been busily "skilling" the client through the consulting project, sometimes the best option is getting an external resource. This is the case when the resources needed to accomplish the objective(s) within the established time line are not available.

Costs Involved. Finally, the action plan includes the total associated costs. The attempt is to make sure that the action plan has a good chance of success. Costing out the project helps avoid moving into a project without the proper resources.

Last, we recommend using a follow-up letter of understanding. This is a letter written by the consultant to the client. The letter should include:

- agreed-on objectives
- specific actions to be taken, by whom, and when
- discussion of the perceived benefits that will occur as a result of the implementation
- discussion of potential negative consequences that could occur as a result of the implementation
- identification of the resources that will be needed to complete the project
- scheduled evaluations by the client as well as the consultant

Exhibit 9 summarizes the action-planning process that we have been discussing.

Action Planning Example

One of the major responsibilities for the nurse consultant in our organization is to enhance knowledge and skill levels of the staff nurses so they can deliver quality care to patients and

Exhibit 9. Action Step Planning Form.

Date:

Project:

Name:

1. State the objective of the action plan in terms of the desired outcomes:

2. List the key tasks, who is responsible for them, and the dates they are to be started and completed:

Key Task   *Responsible Person*   *Start Date*   *End Date*

3. List the key tasks, what material and human resources will be needed, and the projected costs of each:

Key Task   *Materials ($$)*   *Human Resources ($$)*

                    Cost Totals   Cost Totals

---

families. The following is a common experience in the life of the oncology nurse consultant.

Case History. The phone rings, or the beeper beeps. A nurse on the oncology unit is calling the consultant, requesting his or her assistance in teaching a patient to care for his hickman catheter. The oncology nurse consultant (ONC) arranges a time to discuss the situation with the nurse who called (the client).

The meeting takes place with the ONC and the client. The client requests assistance in teaching the patient to care for the catheter at home. The patient is expected to be discharged in four days. The nurse is knowledgeable about the management of the catheter but is unsure about the teaching process, that is, the assessment of the patient's needs. The ONC accepts the consult and enters into a contract. Work now begins on the action plan.

Objective. What is the desired end result? In our situation the desired outcome is for the patient to leave the hospital

Taking Action and Evaluating the Results 149

setting with skills and knowledge on the home care of the hickman catheter. That is the ultimate outcome.

Our more immediate objective is to have the nurse become skilled at doing the necessary patient teaching so we will not be required to continue doing so. The immediate outcome: a nurse skilled in patient education for the care of the hickman.

Listing of Tasks. A specific set of tasks that need to be accomplished are developed. These include:

1. assessment of the nurse to identify the current level of knowledge and skills in the teaching of the patient with regard to the hickman
2. determination of the desired proficiency level for the nurse
3. determination of the information needed for the patient to be considered informed
4. determination of how the nurse will be checked off on the specific tasks

Who Is Responsible? The teaching process involves a joint effort between the ONC and the client. The ONC has responsibility for getting accurate information, and the client has responsibility for learning the details of the information.

For each task it is decided who needs to take the lead. Tasks 1 and 2 are the responsibility of the ONC, tasks 3 and 4 of the ONC and the nurse.

Time Lines. Next, a time line is established for each of the tasks. The total project is assigned a beginning date and an ending date.

Costs: Material and Human Resource Costs. In this example the material costs are minimal, and the human resource costs involve the time of the nurse and the ONC. When projected, the total cost associated with the project is less than sixty dollars.

The above example shows the adaptation of the action plan to the specific needs of the consult. Some consults will be major, for example, the conversion to a new computer system, and others will be minor, for example, the decision to teach a supervisory course. Each will involve a different approach to the action plan. One will require considerable detail and planning, and the other will not.

Computer Assistance

The action plan can be written on paper or computerized. There are a number of project-planning software packages that can be very useful in action planning. Some that we have used include:

1. Who, What, When (WWW). WWW is an easy package to learn and tracks the three major elements—who, what, and when. The software ties these elements together in a daily calendar that tracks the tasks, people, and dates. We have found it to be a very useful management tool for tracking projects. (WWW is developed by Chronos Software, Inc., 1500 Sixteenth St., Ste. 100, San Francisco, Calif. 94103.)

2. Microsoft Project. Microsoft Project is an excellent tool for more complex projects. It allows for detailed tracking of resources needed for action plans. (Microsoft Project is a product of Microsoft Corporation, 16011 NE 36th Way, Redmond, Wash. 98073.)

3. Homemade project planners. The resourceful internal consultant can also use a standard database to develop a shell for tracking a project. This can be an inexpensive but highly useful alternative to commercial packages.

We strongly recommend the use of computers in the action-planning phase. The computer can be a powerful tool and ally in the process of action planning.

Action Planning: Last Thoughts

So far, this chapter has overviewed the details of action planning. The action-planning phase of the consult is important. It provides the structure in which the desired results are

Taking Action and Evaluating the Results 151

achieved. The basis for solid action planning is solid contracting and data collection and analysis.

Evaluation

The next step is evaluation. Evaluation is the means used to determine the value of the consulting project—did we get done what needed to be done in a way that used our resources in an effective and efficient manner? Clients and decision makers in the organization need to know if their investments of time, money, and effort in the consulting project have paid off. Specifically, an evaluation is effective when it determines whether or not the consulting intervention has accomplished the objectives or terms of the contract.

Evaluation is normally thought of as a process that you begin at the end of the project. However, we suggest that evaluation is something that needs to begin early in the life of the project. Objective evaluation requires the identification of criteria and the noting of benchmarks for measurement before the work begins in discussions with the client in the planning phase. Remember, the consultant asked the questions about success: What needs to happen for the project to be successful? What would success look like? What would you not want to happen? These questions will serve the consultant very well as evaluation criteria to measure the degree of success as well as to plan for next steps. Many of us neglect to establish what constitutes success, what it will look like. If we do not take time to define success, we may never know when we successfully achieve our goals.

Evaluation can be a painful and anxiety-producing process. It is often difficult for consultant and client to look critically at what has been accomplished together, especially if all has not gone well (Nadler, 1983, pp. 241–251). For that reason evaluation is frequently not comprehensive or is not done at all. Again, the need to plan for evaluating—to ensure that it will occur in a systematic, objective way—is clear.

As you can see from Figure 16, evaluation is a thread, weaving throughout the entire project. It begins in the contract-

Figure 16. Evaluation: A Time Line.

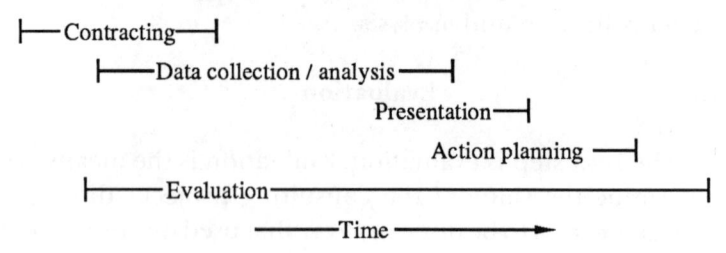

|—Contracting—|
　　|—Data collection / analysis—|
　　　　　　　　　Presentation—|
　　　　　　　　　　　　Action planning —|
|———Evaluation————————————————|
　　　———Time———▶

ing period with questions such as: What is the desired end result? What is the problem that needs to be addressed? It ends in the implementation phase with questions such as: Did we accomplish what we said we would, in the established time frame? What, if anything, still needs to happen?

The purpose of this chapter is to explore the consultant's and client's roles in evaluation. On completion of the chapter you will have an enhanced sense of the importance of the evaluation as the force that drives every phase of the project. You will also be equipped with tools to facilitate the evaluation process.

Purpose of Evaluation

Evaluation is a feedback mechanism indicating the degree of success in meeting the terms of the contract. Windsor and others (1984) cited several purposes for carrying out evaluations. We will translate these into consulting terminology.

1. *Determine the rate and level of attainment of the consulting contract.* We want to determine: Did we get done what needed to get done? To what degree did we accomplish the task? We will look at the outcomes and see what is finished and what left unfinished. As an example, consider a contract we entered into with a client to analyze employee turnover within ten departments and make recommendations for decreasing employee turnover. We miscalculated the time it would take to complete the project and ran three months behind the initially agreed-on

Taking Action and Evaluating the Results 153

time frame. We accomplished the task for several areas, still leaving us with an unfinished part of the contract.

The beautiful part about the consulting process is that solid contracting makes evaluation a "piece of cake." The ongoing contract is the one of the two most important pieces of the consult evaluation. When we ask whether we got done what we wanted to get done, we go back to the contract and see what has happened. In our example, a gross miscalculation was made concerning the time required to collect and analyze the data.

2. *Ascertain the action plan's strengths and weaknesses for making decisions and project planning.* With the action plan we can review specific steps that we took and evaluate the time frame and amount of resources that were used. This gives us a feel for the process that was gone through: Was it an efficient process? Or was it a process that wasted resources? Again, in our turnover example, we did not plan for a workable time frame, and we underestimated the resources required.

3. *Determine the generalization of the overall project or project elements to other departments in the organization.* The consults in which we are involved often have application to other departments as well. If we can develop a good prototype to use with other departments, we will not have to reinvent the wheel. A good example is the turnover work with which we are involved. We are analyzing and predicting employee turnover for a specific department; however, if the process is effective, we will also use it with a number of other departments. The specific questionnaire that we developed, the focus group session, and the analysis of exit interviews are all useful in helping us with our goal for the project—which is effectively analyzing and predicting turnover for the department studied. How will we know if it is successful? Evaluation!

4. *Identify needs or areas that require further work.* There will almost always be some elements left undone at the end of a consult. There may also be new areas to explore. Evaluation provides a tool to say, "We got this much done, and we have these items with which to continue working." This is a powerful function of the evaluation. As we progress with our project on turnover, we are finding that we need to explore one other area,

various position vacancy time frames. We had not considered this aspect in our contracting phase; the client requested our looking into it. In the eyes of our client it was a definite loose end.

5. *Promote positive public relations and organizational awareness.* Organizations need to know what is working. If you show the organization how your consultation is working, the organization will feel better about the dollars that it is spending in your area. Good evaluation provides the organization with signs of accountability.

Our study (Ulschak and SnowAntle, forthcoming) conducted in conjunction with board members of the American Society of Health Education Training found that one key issue identified by respondents was the selection and retention of quality health care employees. With our turnover work the goal is to analyze turnover and make recommendations to decrease turnover within the department under study from an annual percentage of 35 percent to 25 percent. This would translate into major dollar savings to the organization.

In health care organizations it is especially important to show the fruits of your work. That is the way that you continue to justify your existence.

6. *Fulfilling the internal consulting contract.* Evaluation provides a way to close a consult. This is important both psychologically and for good work flow. Psychologically, evaluation provides a closure experience.

Evaluation also concludes the project and means that the work flow can be adjusted to bring in new projects. It represents the ending of the current condition.

Evaluation can be valuable in helping the consultant and the organization to learn from the successes as well as failures. Learning from the mistakes is critical for the organization.

Exhibit 10 provides a hands-on questionnaire for use in evaluation of the project. It will walk through many of the elements that we have been discussing.

Formative and Summative Evaluation

We have essentially been working with two aspects of evaluation: formative and summative. The following sections

Taking Action and Evaluating the Results 155

Exhibit 10. Evaluation Questionnaire.

The purpose of this questionnaire is to walk you through an evaluation process using the contract and action plan. It is a guide that will help you determine if you got done what needed to be done and in an effective manner.

Contract

1. Return to the original contract. What were the presenting problems and issues that needed to be resolved?

2. Complete the following chart for each problem or issue identified during the contracting time.

Problem/Issue   *Desired Outcome*   *Resolved?*

For each "no" under resolved, indicate the next steps to be taken.

3. Were the desired outcomes achieved as a result of the consulting process, or were other factors responsible?

4. If you were to start a similar consult today, what would you do differently to enhance effectiveness and efficiency?

Action Plan

5. List the following components of the action plan:

Issue   *Who Responsible*   *Outcomes*   *Time Frame*   *Cost*

6. Review the list in item 5. Which items were completed?

7. Which items in the list in item 5 were not completed? What needs to happen with each?

Item   *Next Steps*

8. If you were to begin the project today, what would you do differently to enhance the effectiveness and efficiency?

describe both in more detail and review some good questions and thoughts to consider in working with these in a consulting project. Formative evaluation, according to Scriven (1973, p. 60), is used to improve a program while it is still fluid or is still happening by providing feedback to the consultant and client. According to Stufflebeam (1973b, p. 148), the objective with formative or process evaluation is to identify or predict, in process, deficits in the procedural design or its implementation and to maintain a record of procedural events and activities. In the internal consultant model this takes place every step of the way.

Some formative questions include:

- What are the objectives to this point in time, and have we accomplished them?
- Are we still proceeding on our time line?
- What are some of the stumbling blocks, and how are we dealing with them?
- Do we need to make changes in the way the project is being carried out?

Summative evaluation, according to Scriven, is evaluation of a completed product. According to Stufflebeam, the objective of summative or product evaluation is to relate outcome information to objectives. This is the end of the class evaluation—did we pass or not?

Questions to consider here include:

- Was the goal of the contract met?
- What factors determined the success of the project?
- What factors determined the failure of the project?
- What factors contributed to the effectiveness and efficiency of the project?
- What factors subtracted from the effectiveness and efficiency of the project?

Understanding the differences between the two evaluative roles will help the evaluator to delineate the methods that may be appropriately used in the evaluation process.

Taking Action and Evaluating the Results

The method associated with formative evaluation is to (1) monitor the consulting project's procedural barriers and remain alert to unanticipated ones, (2) obtain specified information for programmed decisions, and (3) describe the actual process involved as progress is made through each step of the consulting model.

The method associated with summative evaluation is to (1) define criteria operationally and measure criteria associated with objectives and (2) compare these measurements with predetermined standards, or benchmarks.

Developing Evaluation Designs. The structure of evaluation design is the same for both formative and summative evaluation. The parts include (Stufflebeam, 1973a):

A. *Focusing the evaluation*
  1. The first step is identifying the major level(s) of decision making to be served (for example, departmental, organizational, or community). Try to identify the extent and distribution of the target decision makers — who are you trying to reach? It may start out with a narrow focus such as a single department but often has far-reaching implications for the entire organization.
  2. Next, for each level of decision making, project the decision situations to be served and describe each in terms of its timing, importance, and composition of alternatives.
  3. Define criteria for each decision situation by specifying variables for measurement and standards for use in the judgment of alternatives.
  4. Define policies within which the consultant and client must operate, for example, who will see the data, that bad news will be reported along with the good news, and so on.

B. *Collecting information*
  1. Specify the source of the needed information, for example, records, information from interviews, exit interviews, or personnel files. It is important to establish

access early on and not just assume ready access. This might mean going through an approval process.
2. Specify the instruments and methods for collecting information, for example, survey, observation, or sensing interview. This method will depend very much on what kind of information is needed. If it is factual, we recommend a questionnaire or reports. If you are looking for feelings, opinions, or beliefs, a focus group or one-on-one interview might be best.
3. Specify the sampling procedure to be employed. How will you select a sample, or will you use the entire population? With a large population, using a sample is better. Care must be taken to use a random sample of adequate size for you to generalize your findings back to the population. For example, if you have a population of one hundred, you will probably want a sample size of thirty.
4. Specify conditions for information collection. Individual confidentiality should be respected.
5. Schedule the dates and times for collection of the information. Specify these exactly. The information required is the date, time, who will collect information, and how much time to allow (for example, one hour).

C. *Organizing information*
1. Provide a format for information to be collected, that is, how it will be coded and organized. This becomes extremely important when you are using large groups or several different groups.
2. Data can be organized according to the group, or it may be based on another variable such as professional group, age, educational preparation, or length of tenure. It really depends on the individual project and the purpose behind collecting the information.

D. *Analyzing information*
1. Select the statistical/analytical procedures to be employed. This procedure will depend on what questions you want answered and what kinds of data you have collected (qualitative or quantitative). The statistics

Taking Action and Evaluating the Results

most commonly used are the mean and standard frequency counts. When we want to do more sophisticated comparisons, we move into correlational analysis; when we have several variables to compare, we use multivariate analysis. Ask yourself, "What questions do I need answered?" Then collect the types of data that will help answer these questions and select a statistical method appropriate for use with your data type.

E. *Reporting information*
   1. Define the audience for the evaluation report. Who will be receiving the information? Who are the clients and key decision makers? Essentially, this should have already been established in the contract, so check it.
   2. Specify the means for report delivery. How will you deliver? What types of AV handouts will you use? How long will the presentation be?
   3. Specify type format for the evaluation report. Are you looking at a three-page or a thirty-page report? Remember—keep it lean and mean. Executive summaries at the beginning are helpful.
   4. Schedule the report meeting(s). Make sure that those attending know when, where, how long, and the purpose of meeting and why they are included.

F. *Administering evaluation*
   1. Define material and human resources required and the plan for meeting these requirements—for example, who needs to be involved, other material and equipment needed, and length of time.
   2. Evaluate the design for providing information that is valid, reliable, credible, and timely. This ties us back to methods for collection and a time frame for completion.
   3. Specify and schedule means for periodic updating of the evaluation design:
      a. How will you accomplish "midterm" checks?
      b. What are indicators that things are going well or not well?

            c. How will you notify others of progress and any changes?
G. *Determining associated costs*
    1. The design and analysis of the evaluation are time-consuming and complex. However, they are essential in guiding the consultant and client along each phase of the consulting model, the assessment, planning implementation, and evaluation. The goal is to obtain adequate information to support vital decision making.
H. *Using outside evaluators*
    1. There are some occasions when an outside evaluator may be very useful. Sometimes the issues may be too sensitive for the internal consultant, and the organization needs an outside objective opinion. Another occasion to use an external consultant is when the internal consultant does not have the necessary skills or expertise to complete the project. Sometimes when immediate results are needed, an external is more able to focus on only the project at hand, whereas the internal consultant is trying to juggle ten other projects.

Evaluation Walk-Through

As mentioned, we have been involved in a turnover study in the organization. There has been some high turnover in a few departments, and we were called in to review the situation and give recommendations based on our findings. We will continue to use this example to assist us in outlining a walk-through of the evaluation process.

1. Focusing the Evaluation. The client was the associate administrator, and he had initiated the consult with us. Our report would go to him. However, due to the nature of the issue, other key decision makers would also be served. These were the executive director, director of human resources, and department director.

2. Collecting Information. Information would be collected from a variety of sources. We arrived at the following:

Taking Action and Evaluating the Results

Event
1. Focus groups
2. Exit interview records
3. Telephone survey
4. Record information
5. Questionnaire survey

Dates: March 2, 3, 4

Time: 1:00 P.M.

Who involved: Three groups of eight department workers

How information collected: Focus group and questionnaire

Who collects information: Consultants

Cost: Total cost was three hundred dollars, including both human resources and material costs (employees' time, facilitator's time, development costs, paper costs, AV use).

Time frame: One hour each (three hours total) for the focus group sessions. Other time included five hours for telephone surveys and five hours for obtaining information from exit interviews and other reports.

3. Organizing Information. We organized the information according to the groups and variables involved such as length of tenure, job satisfaction, and the intent to stay on the job. We selected these variables because they are strong predications of turnover.

4. Analyzing Information. We entered the data into the computer and then analyzed them using information collected on the turnover variables. At that time we did a comparison using a discriminate function analysis to compare employees who had quit to those who stayed.

5. Reporting Information. The ten-page report was presented to the associate administrator and was then presented in detail in a group meeting with the other key decision makers. Overheads and a flip chart were used as tools to facilitate presenting the information.

162 **Consultation Skills for Health Care Professionals**

Exhibit 11. Action-Planning and Evaluation Skills Checklist.

Action Planning and Evaluation
__ 1. Ability to develop an action plan consisting of who, what, when, where, why, how much, and the desired outcomes
__ 2. Ability to monitor and track the progress of an action plan
__ 3. Ability to respond to changes and make midcourse corrections
__ 4. Ability to control anxiety while in the midst of a consultation
__ 5. Ability to design forms and inventories to aid in an evaluation
__ 6. Ability to feel comfortable with the client's review of your work
__ 7. Ability to terminate and have closure with a project

6. Administering Evaluation. This was the time that next steps were introduced along with material and human resources to meet the requirements. A schedule was presented for who, what, when, where, how, and the midcheck evaluation:

Recommendation: To review current orientation program and make recommendations to increase its effectiveness.

Time to start: May 7

End date: May 20

Who: Consultants, department director

Resources: Human and material resources include facilitator's time for preparing and implementing the sessions, the analysis of salary for positions and the development of a career ladder, and AV materials (overheads, flip charts).

Cost: $190

This walk-through provides a quick overview of the evaluation process. Take the steps and fit them to your needs and situation.

Exhibit 11 is a final self-check list to aid the internal consultant in determining his or her degree of readiness in implementing this phase of the project.

Some Final Thoughts: Termination

Throughout this book we have been describing the consult as a relationship between a helpee and a helper. Much effort

Taking Action and Evaluating the Results

was put into the building of the relationship between the client and the consultant in order to successfully work together to meet the terms of the contract. On project completion, deliberate attention needs to be focused on bringing closure.

There are three situations involving closure. The first is when the client wants to terminate the project prematurely. Perhaps the heat gets turned up. The second is when the time is right for the termination of the project, and the project was not successful. The third is when the project is completed, and it has been a success. Let us take a look at each.

The premature closure often occurs when things start to get a little bumpy. The client feels the pressure of change and wants a quick fix. Or maybe the client realizes that there is no quick fix. The intervention suggested by the consultant may seem to make things worse rather than better—remember the change cycle from Chapter One? One thing that frequently happens is that things do get worse before they get better.

The appropriate termination here is to go back and review the contract. There needs to be a "time out." The consultant's role is to help with the termination of the relationship in such a way that there is damage control on the part of the client. The goal is to leave the relationship as solid as possible. This means making a list of the things done and the things left undone. It is very important to be clear about the work that is left.

We recently had a client decide to quit halfway through a project, and our role became helping the client do this in a way that "saved face." We helped explore the options and the consequences of making the decision to close down the process.

The second scenario is shutting down an unsuccessful project. This is a difficult process. Our experience is that what is needed on everyone's part is honesty. The most important part of the process is to be open to the fact that we did not accomplish what we wanted to accomplish. Significant learnings often occur in this type of setting, and the way to those learnings is through the experience of being honest about what failed.

The last scenario is ending the successful project. Again, it is important that the parties involved are honest with the

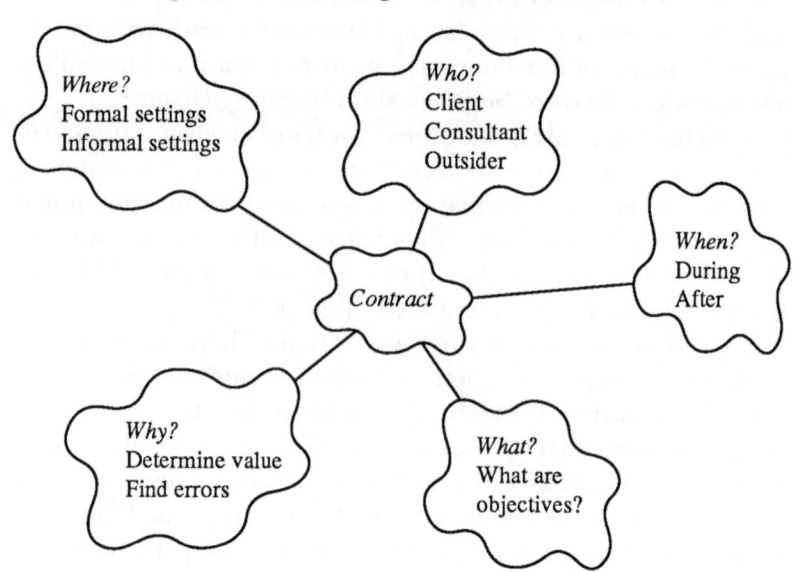

164 Consultation Skills for Health Care Professionals

Figure 17. Contracting: The Core of Evaluation.

- **Where?** Formal settings / Informal settings
- **Who?** Client / Consultant / Outsider
- **When?** During / After
- **Why?** Determine value / Find errors
- **What?** What are objectives?
- *Contract*

outcomes and their excitement about the success and, for you the consultant, that you make sure that the client feels the ownership of success. The client is the winner along with yourself. We believe that there is an "art of celebration" and that the consultant and the client need to participate in that art.

In all cases, the termination of the relationship needs to celebrate the successful parts of the consultation, identify clearly the sense of loss and failure with the unsuccessful parts, and say good-bye to this particular contract. It is only through saying good-bye that the consultant will be ready for the next consultation and the client ready for the next consultant.

Conclusion

This chapter has been about action plans and evaluation. Our thesis is that the action plan is one of the structures of effective consultations. The action plan takes an idea and implements it. It makes things happen.

Evaluation is the dessert after the meal. It lets us know

Taking Action and Evaluating the Results

how we have done. It provides us with the feedback about the good news and the bad news of what we have been about. As Figure 17 indicates, it is driven by the contract. So, we come full circle—in the beginning was the contract, and we now come back to the contract to decide our final evaluation.

III

Becoming an Effective Internal Consultant

III

Becoming an Effective
Internal Consultant

8

Understanding the Culture of the Organization

Think about your present organization. What are some unstated rules of conduct? What are some unstated expected behaviors that would get you in deep trouble should you violate them? What are some ways of getting work done that are unique to your setting and your organization?

Now think about a previous organization of which you have been part. What were some of the unstated rules of conduct in that organization? What were some of the expected behaviors, and what would happen if you were to violate them?

These questions begin to get at the topic of organizational culture. Each organization has a unique culture. It is their "fingerprint." For some organizations that fingerprint is clear and distinct, and for other organizations it is hazy and unclear. Nevertheless the fingerprint is there.

Why is it important for the internal consultant to have an understanding of and respect for culture? Quite simply, the organizational culture will provide the limits of the internal consultant's effectiveness. Internal consulting depends on the flow of information from one person to another. Organizational cultures define the formal and informal norms for behavior that determine what kinds of information can be shared and in what kind of settings. The culture defines what leadership means, how decisions will get made, what problem-solving behaviors are acceptable, how conflicts between individuals and departments will be handled, and, in general, how the organization will go about its business. Take problem solving, for example. In one organizational culture problem solving will be encouraged at all levels. In another organization managers will be careful to keep "their cards close to their vest" and not to admit problems or failures because to do so in their culture would mean a loss of status and even loss of job.

Organizational culture, then, provides the context for the work of the internal consultant. The more the internal consultant is aware of the culture and its strengths and limitations, the better the internal consultant will be in working effectively within the culture. The internal consultant's role is to work within the culture while at the same time recognizing some of that culture's limitations.

The purpose of this chapter is to (1) define culture and discuss some of the implications of the definition, (2) identify ways to identify organizational culture, and (3) suggest ways for the internal consultant to be sensitive to culture and overcome cultural barriers.

However, we want to start with a model for viewing organizations. Ulschak (1988, pp. 6–29) provides one model for viewing organizations. Too often the internal consultant focuses on a small portion of the organization when there is a need to look at the broader organization. Our model will provide a broader view.

Organizational Overview

We have found the CPR + F model simple yet effective for looking at organizations. Consider the view of the organization as shown using that model in Figure 18.

The model has a series of concentric circles. The center circle is the purpose. The components of purpose are the value core of the organization, mission, goals, and objectives. The purpose is the core of what the organization is about. It is the

Understanding the Culture of the Organization 171

Figure 18. CPR + F Model: The Organization.

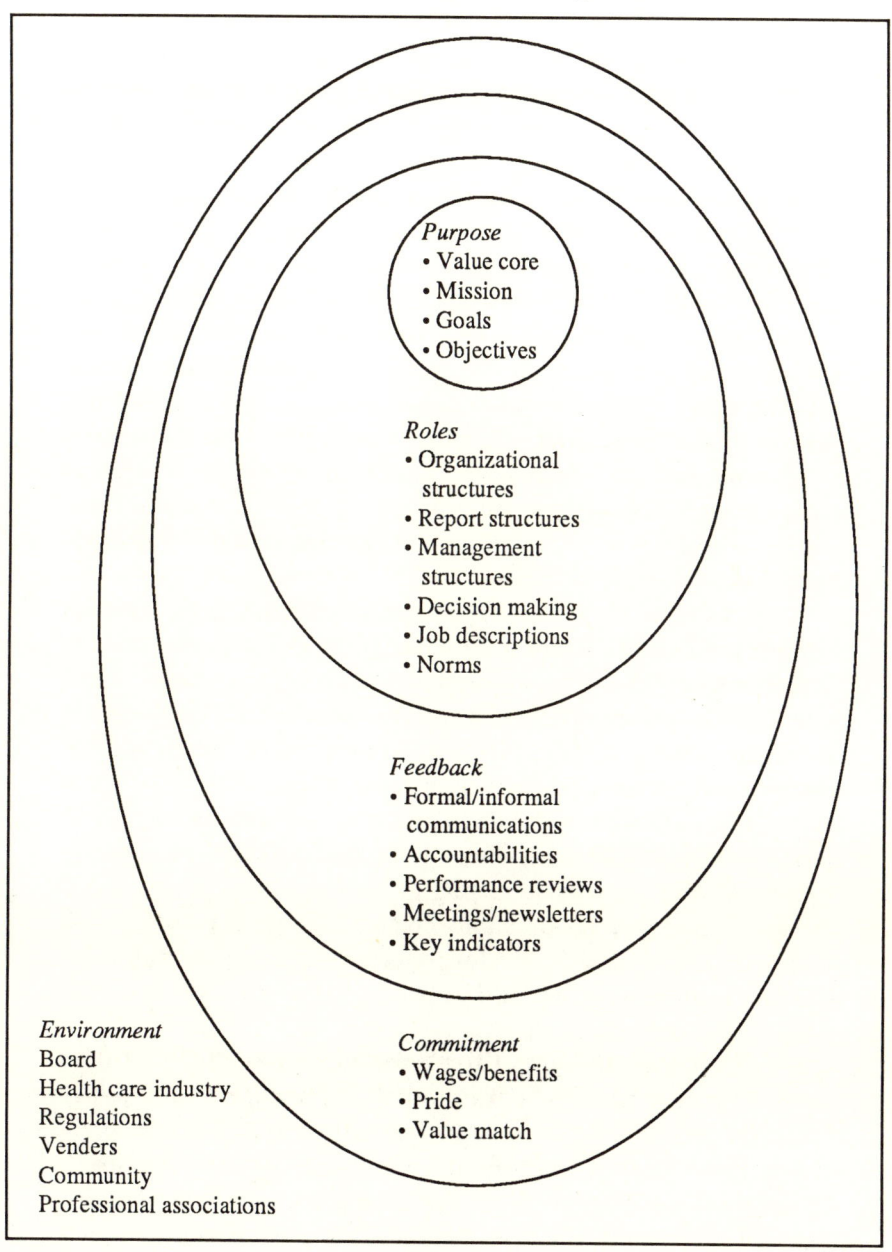

Purpose
- Value core
- Mission
- Goals
- Objectives

Roles
- Organizational structures
- Report structures
- Management structures
- Decision making
- Job descriptions
- Norms

Feedback
- Formal/informal communications
- Accountabilities
- Performance reviews
- Meetings/newsletters
- Key indicators

Environment
Board
Health care industry
Regulations
Venders
Community
Professional associations

Commitment
- Wages/benefits
- Pride
- Value match

Culture

organization's direction. The remaining circles revolve around the purpose.

The next circle out is roles. This includes the organizational structure, report structures, management structures, decision making, norms, and job descriptions. It includes those components of the organization that define the roles and relationships of people in the organization. It is a definition of the work flow and the relation of work flow to the organization. Again, the elements that define the role need to be in line with the organization's core purpose.

The next circle out is feedback. Feedback systems in the organization include such things as the internal communications, formal and informal communications, accountabilities, meetings and newsletters, performance reviews, key financial indicators, and various reports that let members know what is happening in the organization and is of concern for the individual. The feedback provides the organization with information about votes and purpose.

The next circle, which encompasses the first three, is commitment. Commitment is what fuels the organization. It includes such things as personal satisfactions, wages and salary plans, pride, job enrichments, and the value match between the individual and the organization. Commitment builds on the clarity of the other parts of the organization.

The last circle is the environment in which the organization finds itself. This consists of the health care trends, regulatory bodies, boards, licensing groups, venders, professional associations, and so on. The circles fall in a box labeled "culture." The sum of the circles generates the corporate culture. Culture is the environment that provides the context for all the work of the organization.

What does this model do for the internal consultant? Most important, it provides a framework for thinking about the broader context of the consult. Remember our discussion regarding the client? The ultimate client is the organization itself. When we are working in a portion of a department or a department in the organization, we need to be sensitive to the impact of our work on the overall organization. Health care organiza-

Understanding the Culture of the Organization 173

tions are highly complex, and changes in one part may mean changes in other parts. Changing the procedures in how a lab workup is done impacts others in the organization. The value of the organizational model is that it enables the internal consultant to think about how the current consult is impacting the overall purpose, roles, commitment, and feedback systems in the organization. And the context of all organization is its culture.

What Is Culture?

What is culture?

This simple analogy can be useful in understanding organizational culture. Imagine that you are traveling in a foreign country. You are alert to the difference in language, dress, money, customs, and so on. The people you meet are different from you, and they do things differently than you are used to doing them. Their language is different. Their money is different. Their clothes are different. Their food is different. These are the visible parts of the culture. These are the "clothes" the culture puts on for others. This is the surface of the culture.

One layer beneath this surface are the norms that govern the behaviors of the individuals in that culture. Norms are the accepted and expected ways of behaving. There are norms regarding how individuals will behave toward one another, how conflict is managed, how children get raised, family expectations, what role work has in life, and the like. The norms are the "rules" that govern how the people will relate to one another in that culture.

However, beneath those surface items are the assumptions and values that culture has regarding life and the best way to approach life. There are values regarding how individuals are to relate to others. There are values about conflict and how it is to be managed. There are values about the importance of the individual, family, and work. The values are under the norms, which are under the visual trappings of the culture. It is the values and the assumptions that are the driving force of the culture. They are less obvious to the casual observer, but they are

Figure 19. The Iceberg Model of Corporate Culture.

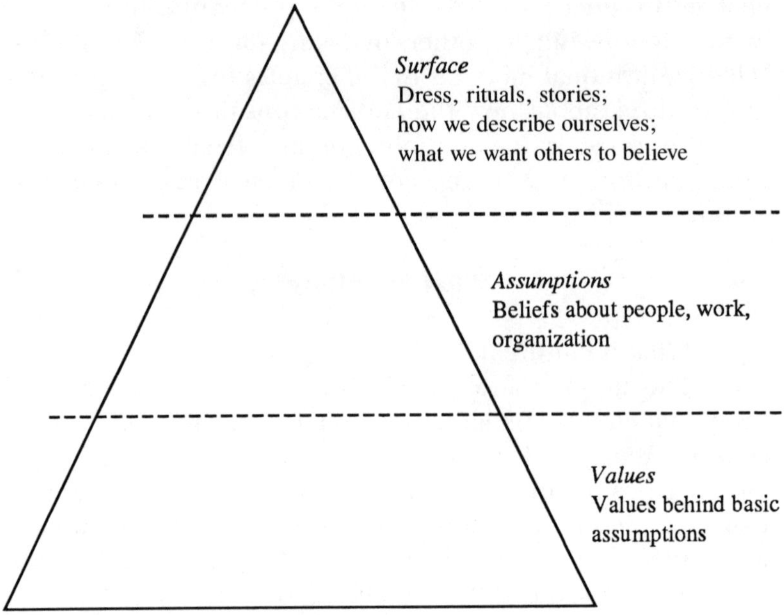

Surface
Dress, rituals, stories;
how we describe ourselves;
what we want others to believe

Assumptions
Beliefs about people, work, organization

Values
Values behind basic assumptions

Source: Ulschak, 1989.

there and are the culture's driving force. Figure 19 graphically illustrates the cultural layers.

Traveling in different countries provides one example of culture. Another example of culture can be found in a single country or single city. A friend relates the example of growing up in a rural midwestern area and then moving to an urban area. He describes the difference between rural hospitality and urban hospitality. For example, he remembers driving down the roads in western North Dakota and coming across a stalled motorist. The rural hospitality was to stop and help. That was the expected behavior, and any less was unacceptable. However, when he moved to the city, the definition changed. The first time he ran across a stranded motorist in the city and stopped to help, he realized that he had become more of a traffic hazard than a help. The two areas simply have different ways of doing things. Different areas of the country have different cultures in the larger culture.

Understanding the Culture of the Organization 175

The same is true in organizations. Organizations have their own culture—their own way of doing things. A definition that we like to use for organizational culture comes from Edgar Schein (1985, p. 9):

> A pattern of basic assumptions—invented, discovered, or developed by a given group as it learns to cope with its problems of external adaptation and internal integration—that worked well enough to be considered valid and therefore, to be taught to new members as the correct way to perceive, think, and feel in relation to those problems.

The definition has several important implications. Each of these will be discussed in some detail.

Culture is a learned "pattern of basic assumptions." First of all, culture is learned basic assumptions. Culture does not just happen; it is developed and solidified over time. In the last part of this chapter we will discuss the life cycle of an organization and present one way of thinking about an organization's life and death. Having been part of the start-up of a new organization, we are keenly aware of how culture is learned. There is the influence of those who wanted to bring the organization into existence and their values about work and health care. There is the influence of those who were hired to develop the departments in the organization. There is the learning from experience what works and does not work.

All of these learnings become the assumptions of the culture. These assumptions become the foundation for expectations of behavior. For example, in the start-up organization of which we were part, the founding director was a man very influenced by customer service and guest relations. He hired people of like mind and developed a culture that had guest relations as a core set of assumptions. Guest relations became a key component of orientation, a part of the reward system for individual performance, and a part of the annual organizational objectives. More important, a guest relations norm developed. If an employee was walking down the hall and observed a person who appeared lost, it was expected that the employee would approach the individual and offer help. This is a learned norm. And, once learned, the norm drops out of consciousness and simply becomes an expectation.

A good example of assumptions is the classic managerial work of Douglas McGregor (1957) and the identification of the conventional view and the "new theory." The conventional view (Theory X) had some of these as its basic assumptions:

1. The average person is by nature lazy and works as little as possible.
2. The average person lacks ambition and prefers to be led.
3. The average person is self-centered and does not care about the organizational needs.
4. The average person is by nature resistant to change.

The new theory (Theory Y) had some of these as its basic assumptions:

1. The average person is not passive or resistant to the organizational needs. That is a result of experience in organizations.
2. The average individual has within himself or herself the ability for self-motivation and the ability to assume responsibility. Management's role is to assist that development.
3. Management's role is to arrange organizational conditions such that individuals can achieve their goals best by working toward the organizational goals.

Think for a moment about these two sets of assumptions. Our role is not to say yes or no to McGregor regarding them but to think about the implications of each for the work force. The two theories represent two distinct sets of assumptions that will generate different sets of management behaviors and result in different organizational cultures.

Think about doing consulting work in a department that believes that people are naturally lazy, lack ambition, need to be

Understanding the Culture of the Organization 177

watched, and do not care about the organization. How will that impact your internal consultant role?

Now think about doing consulting work in a department that believes that people are self-motivated and can take responsibility, people are not passive, and management's role is to arrange conditions so the people can achieve both organizational and personal goals. How will that impact your internal consultant role?

Now, think about your current organization. What are some key assumptions that form the basis of your culture? How do these impact the way you do internal consulting?

The first important point is: culture is a set of assumptions that are learned and expected.

"Invented...by a given group as it learns to cope with its problems of external adaptation and internal integration..." The work of all organizations has two elements. The first element is getting the work done. This is the internal structure, the reward systems, the work flow, and all the other components so important in internally organizing the organization.

The second element is the organization's business. This is the products produced, marketing efforts, getting in the client, and general mission of the organization. For health care organizations it is the services provided, the market shares of types of services, the profits returned on the services, and so on.

The organizational culture defines both elements. It determines the type of ethic that the organization has as it approaches the internal organizing and the external business.

The internal organization of the organization cannot exist without the business of the organization, and the business makes no sense without the internal organization. They are symbiotic.

The role of the internal consultant is to work with both the internal integration and the external adaptation. For example, working with a department on its work flow is an example of internal integration. The internal consultant is working with the department to increase its work-flow effectiveness. The internal consultant working with a department regarding a new product will be working with the interface between the organization and the environment.

While most of the internal consultant's work relates to internal integration, there is some work that relates to the external adaptation. Try to think of some internal consulting projects in your organization that mainly deal with internal integration and some that mainly deal with external adaptation.

"Worked well enough...to be taught to new members." Culture is learned from what works. The internal consultant must realize this. The culture is there because it has assisted the organization in survival. Therefore, changes that are perceived to impact the culture are not taken lightly. It means the organization itself will resist any attempt to challenge one of its core beliefs. The internal consultant who suddenly finds himself in the middle of a conflict over what he considers a minor change is probably being perceived as challenging one of those core assumptions. He may be told, "It's worked well in the past—don't change it."

The important point, one we discussed in Chapter One, is that change that appears to challenge the core culture is not going to be successful. Just as an individual who has learned a certain way of relating will not readily change that way of relating even when it no longer works, the same is true of the organization.

One last point. The learnings of the culture are significant enough that they are taught to new persons coming into the organization. That is critical, and it places a new emphasis on orientation. Orientation is not just an exercise in putting people through the mandated programs of the organization (for example, fire and safety, personnel regulations, infection control, and so on). It is a vital time of introducing the new members of the organization to the culture.

What are some ways that new people coming into your organization learn the key assumptions you identified earlier? Where did you learn them when you came into the organization?

The above, then, represent some aspects of organizational culture. There are a few other points we want to make regarding

Understanding the Culture of the Organization 179

organizational culture that are also important for the internal consultant. These points are:

1. Culture is relatively transparent to its members.
2. Cultures are changing and dynamic.
3. Cultures contain subcultures.
4. No one culture is best for all organizations.
5. Not all cultural changes are equally important.
6. Awareness of corporate culture makes good business sense.

First, the assumptions of the organizational culture are transparent to the organization. Once learned, they become taken for granted. Think about this for a moment.

My own culture is transparent to me. I see through it. Why? Because I have grown to expect that certain things are done in certain ways. I have grown to expect them. Once I have grown to expect them, I "forget" them. That is why it is typically difficult to get at an organizational culture by asking the question: What is your culture? Culture is like water to a fish or air to a bird—it is simply there. It is expected.

This transparent quality of culture has special implications for the internal consultant. First, the consultant is part of the culture—the culture will be transparent to the consultant as well as the client. This will be discussed more later.

Second, cultures are dynamic and changing. Think about your health care organization in the last few years. Certainly the impact on changing health care reimbursement has meant significant cultural change for many organizations. Organizations that were in the health care business to take care of the sick and needy suddenly found that their primary mission was being challenged by another agenda—the business side of the organization, which called for making a profit.

The dynamic quality of culture means that it is both a process and a product. The process quality means that culture is continually evolving. Again, we can look at health care in the past few years and see how the culture of health care organizations has evolved. Cultures have changed in response to the environmental change. The product side is what we look for when we say, "What is the culture of this organization?" We are looking at the culture for that moment in time. This demands flexibility of the internal consultant.

Third, cultures contain subcultures that can either contribute to the work of the organization or subtract from it. Think about your organization. Do you notice a difference in "culture" as you go from department to department? Or in a specific department do you have a sense of the subgroups in it?

The subcultures in health care organizations are obvious at times. Think of the operating room. They have their own dress, environment, rules of conduct, and so on. They even have big signs on the doors that say: "Authorized Personnel Only." Think of the culture of the critical care area or emergency room and compare that to a medical unit. Then think about the world of the lab, radiology, pharmacy, business office, or administration. Each has its own unique culture.

The first problem is identifying the subcultures. The next problem is evaluating if that subculture contributes to or subtracts from the overall culture.

Fourth, no one culture is best for all health care organizations. The search for the "holy grail of health care cultures" is in vain. Barney (1986, p. 656) provides an excellent discussion that it is precisely the uniqueness of a successful corporate culture that makes it difficult to imitate. If the successful culture were readily imitated, everyone would do it. The real issue becomes how to build the unique culture of the specific organization of which we are part.

Fifth, not all cultural elements are equally important. Some are vital to the workings of the organization, and others are nice but not necessary. This is important for the internal consultant to know. She needs to know if the project she is working on has major organizational sensitivities or if it is minor to the working of the organization. One way to learn which is by doing something and observing the organization's reaction.

Sixth, being aware of corporate culture makes good business sense. The internal consultant needs to have such an awareness. Corporate culture impacts the total working of the

Understanding the Culture of the Organization 181

organization. Therefore, spending time to become aware of culture's impact makes good business sense no matter what kind of internal consulting I am doing.

Organizational culture sets the rules for the game of internal consulting. The next section will take this thought a step further and discuss the implications for the internal consultant.

Keys for the Internal Consultant

Why is understanding culture important for the internal consultant? The response is simple: culture provides the limits of what the internal consultant can do. In this section we will focus on some major implications for the internal consultant in problem solving, organizational subculture, and the consulting role and consulting process.

Problem Solving. The primary relationship of the internal consultant to the client is that of helper to helpee. One important implication of culture for the internal consultant is that of defining what helping and being helped mean in the organization.

Remember the earlier discussion regarding first-degree, second-degree, and third-degree problems? Another set of questions precede determining the degree of a problem. Organizations have "permissions" that must be considered. Some of these are:

1. Is it permissible to have problems? Some organizations do not think so. This may be articulated as something like: "We want solutions, not problems." The implication is not to bring up problems. This invites an organization where individuals are oblivious to problems. Most organizations say they want to take risks, identify problems, and so on. The key is to determine whether the organization actually lives that out or instead attaches some type of punishment to having problems.

2. Is it permissible to identify problems? Some organizations do not reward individuals for identifying problems. You can tell that by simply asking around. Ask a few employees what

happens to people who identify problems. Are they rewarded for diligence or punished for stupidity? In the latter case, problems are swept under the rug. Naturally, this creates a rather lumpy rug. The sense is to avoid the problems and ignore their presence. Eventually, the problems will make themselves known, and then the organization will have to recognize them to some degree. This is known as crisis management. Such an organization will be in crisis a good deal of the time.

3. Is it permissible to solve problems? Other organizations appear to be stuck and cannot seem to get beyond the identification of problems. Is the resolution of problems really valued by the culture? Or is the problem resolution ignored? Some organizations will put roadblocks in the way of problem resolution, even though they claim to want that resolution.

The internal consultant must be sensitive to the organization's beliefs about identifying and resolving problems and then work with these assumptions. Some useful questions are:

1. What happens to people who identify problems in this organization? Are they successful or not?
2. Is it okay to ask for assistance in resolving issues? Or is this seen as weakness?
3. How do problems finally get resolved? If an audit trail is attached to a problem, where does it go, and when does it get resolved?
4. Am I welcomed in departments, or do they want to meet with me "after midnight" and when no one else is around to see?
5. How often are my views of the total organization asked for by others in the organization?

Organizational Subcultures. Organizations have subcultures that may or may not be in line with the overall organization. The three types are:

1. The subculture is in line with the organizational culture. The subculture is on purpose with the total organization.
2. The subculture is not in line with the organization but does

Understanding the Culture of the Organization 183

not detract from it and in some cases may add to the organization. A good example is "skunk works." (Skunk works are subunits of an organization that are given a license to go and create outside of the mainstream organization. In this setting the subculture is not necessarily on purpose, but it is not a negative force.)
3. The subculture is counter to the organization and actually detracts from it.

The internal consultant must deal with this third type of subculture very sensitively. Why? There may be some ethical considerations in working with the counterculture. If it is going in ways that deliberately are not positive for the organization, the consultant's role should not be to strengthen it. In addition, the internal consultant may find himself in a major political pinch. The primary question for the internal consultant will be: How do I assist this department in getting back on purpose with the organization?

What does this mean for the internal consultant? First, it is useful for the internal consultant to be sensitive to departmental differences and how these differences fit into the overall culture. Part of this sensitivity concerns survival because the internal consultant may get caught in between. Second, the subculture will impact how the internal consultant goes about his or her work. The consulting process may need to be modified in working with different subcultures.

Impact on the Role. How does culture impact on the four major internal consultant roles we discussed? The questions in the decision tree are impacted by culture. For example, some cultures will operate with perpetual time crunches. In such a department the internal consultant can expect that much of the time he or she will be called in to do "fire fighting." Most projects will involve some type of crisis.

Obviously, the presence of trust is a significant cultural element. Does the culture support and enhance trust? Why is that important? Trust is important because of the flow of information. Without trust the flow of information can be minimal.

One impact of culture on the consultant's role, then, is the effect the culture has on the elements in the decision tree. In general, the more a culture restricts the flow of information, the more the internal consultant will lean toward the roles of director and counselor because of the lack of information. Facilitation becomes meaningless because there is simply no information flowing in the organization.

If part of the consult role is to do team building, the facilitator role becomes a role for building trust in the department. Otherwise this role is limited.

Impact on Consulting Process. If we view the consulting process as feeding on valid information and information flow, the key question that needs to be asked regarding cultural impact on the consulting process is: Does the culture support the flow of valid information or not? If not, how do I compensate for the information?

Information flow is key at all phases of the consulting process. Contracting is a dead end if valid information is not part of the process. Data collection and analysis are futile if valid information cannot be tapped into. Presentations will miss the critical elements without the flow of information. The impact of culture on action planning and evaluation is equally great.

One area of culture, then, is its impact on the availability of valid information. We could look at the Theory X and Theory Y approaches to people and discuss their implications for each stage of the consulting process. However, the critical factor is that of the flow of information. That is the lifeblood of the consultation process.

Identifying Organizational Culture

The question for the internal consultant is: How do I go about identifying the culture in which I am so I can determine some of the impacts it is having on me?

There are several possible tools. This section will suggest a number of them. However, remember that the culture is difficult to get a handle on. Culture is dynamic, and parts of it are

Understanding the Culture of the Organization   185

changing. This means that you have to be sensitive to the change and be ready to redefine culture.

Here are some specific strategies for identifying your organizational culture:

1. The times of greatest sensitivity to culture are on entry to the organization, when leaving the organization, and during organizational transitions. One strategy is to ask people who are just coming into the organization what they see in it. What are some of the similarities and differences between here and their last organization? What do they notice about people? The way work is organized? The sensitivity to the work environment?

Also, when people are leaving the organization, take them to coffee and ask them about what they have experienced. What makes a person a success in this organization? A failure? What are the expected norms? What does it take to get fired?

Finally, when the organization is in the middle of significant change, ask questions about what people are experiencing and seeing. What does the change mean? What will they lose and gain from it?

As discussed earlier, this is detective work. It involves asking lots of questions and listening to responses and then beginning to make sense of the responses.

2. Work joint projects with outside consultants when possible. This is an excellent place to pick up the outsider's point of view. When we work jointly with external consultants, we like to pick them up from and drive them to the airport; we frequently learn much about what the consultant has seen in our organization in this time span. Ask the consultant questions such as: What stands out for you about our organization? What are similarities and differences you see with us compared to other organizations of which you are part? What are key organizational issues for you?

It is important to weight the responses. The consultant may have a vested interest in responding in a certain way. If the consultant sees this as an opportunity for additional work, she or he may filter some of the comments. However, as we discussed earlier, one of the most effective consulting teams is that of an external and internal consultant working together.

We have recently been working with an external consultant hired to work with the board. The relationship has been outstanding because we have built on the strengths of having both an external and an internal consultant. The external person has all the advantages of being external. We have all the advantages of being internal. Because we are sensitive and intentional with each other, the project has been greatly enhanced. When the external person leaves the organization, we will be wiser, and there will be more skills in our organization.

3. Take time to review what the organization says about itself. Read the mission statement, goals, employee newsletter, and so on. What does this organization say about itself in print? This reveals the espoused culture, that is, the culture the organization wants to project to the world. There can be good learnings about what the culture wants others to believe. What are the themes that consistently get addressed? What are the standard publications? What are the standard stories? For example, are the stories regarding patient care, research, or education? Or some combination of these? Make a listing of themes from the story.

Also, be sensitive to the cosmetic appearance of the publications. The cosmetics are a story in and of itself. Are the publications professionally done? What is the quality of the articles?

4. Take time and walk through the organization. What do you see? Imagine that you are an outsider walking through the organization. What do you hear? See? Feel? Smell? As you tour, what do you see as you pass through various departments? How are you greeted? Is the work area comfortably messy, or is it completely clean? Do the workers appear friendly, or are they stressed out? What kind of wall hangings are there? What does this say about the department? Walk out of the building and come back in. What is your first impression? Again, simply make note of things that you see.

5. Imagine that your organization is a family. What kind of family is it? Who are the parents of this family? Think about specific persons when you answer this. What does the family

Understanding the Culture of the Organization

want to say to the world? What does the family say internally to itself? What are some of the family secrets?

6. Use questionnaires and interviews. In a previous chapter we discussed a number of methods for gathering information. Take some of those techniques and apply them to identification of culture.

The above are some useful ways for getting at the culture of an organization or simply a department. The important point is that the internal consultant needs to be continually aware of the cultural context and how the work that he or she is doing is impacted by and impacting that culture.

You might keep a notebook of cultural learnings and update it from time to time with new observations. In the same way a tourist visiting another culture makes notes about the "interesting and strange habits and behaviors of the natives," make notes about your organization.

Organizational Culture Life Cycle

Organizations change. Organizational cultures change. We know this, and yet there is a tendency to forget it until there are radical changes. We believe that it is important for the internal consultant to be aware of the stages of the organizational life cycle, just as a psychologist or psychiatrist needs to have basic knowledge of human development.

There are a number of models for the organizational life cycle. The one that we have found most useful is that of Adizes (1988), shown in Figure 20.

The foundation of Adizes's model is that effective organizations have four key characteristics. First, they produce results. Without results they do not stay in business. This is the P part of the model. A strong P means that there is a primary emphasis on results and efficient achievement of results in the organization.

Second, they administer resources effectively. This means they use the resources, both human and financial, wisely. This is the A in the model. A strong A means that the administrative side of the organization is strong. It has policies and procedures

Figure 20. Adizes Model.

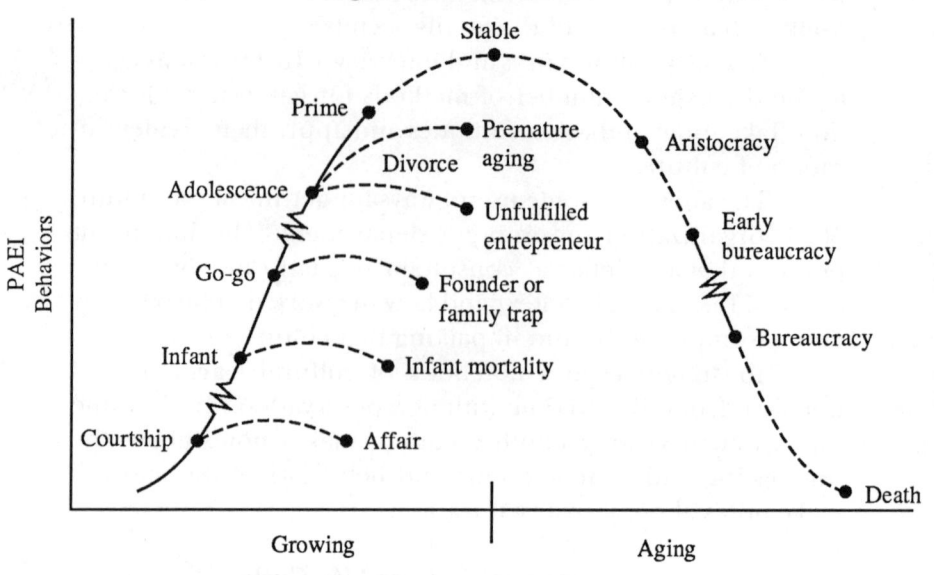

Source: Adizes, 1988. Used with permission.

that must be followed. Decisions must be made in the right sequence with the right timing.

Third, they are entrepreneurial. They respond to environmental changes. This is the E of the model. The focus is on adaptive changes, and the organization is into risk taking and creativity.

Fourth, they integrate functions. They communicate what is going on between the members of the organization. This is the I of the model. The organization is strong in building the team and integrating the efforts of all parts of the organization.

In the life cycle model of the organization, the first half of the organization's life is an ascending curve. The general principles are that (1) everything is permitted unless it is forbidden, (2) there is a lot of entrepreneurial spirit, and (3) there is a lot of energy in the organization. Next, the organizational curve is descending. Typically, the organization grows in bureaucracy. The administrative function dominates, and everything is for-

Understanding the Culture of the Organization 189

bidden unless it is permitted. These patterns are mapped in Figure 20.

The stages of the organizational life cycle become:

A. Ascending curve
    1. Courtship. Courtship is the time when there is no organization. It is a time of dreams about the organization. It needs a strong E function to do the dreaming and speculating. Typically, this is a time of excitement and promise and frantic activity. In our work with start-up organizations, we have found that this is a very exciting time for people. There is a missionary zeal about the organization. The dysfunction during this time period is known as an "affair." The commitment level of the founders is miniscule. At the sign of danger, the commitment evaporates.
    2. Infancy. During infancy the key for the organization is producing results. It has been birthed, and now the challenge is to produce results. During this phase the dreamers are discouraged. The members of the organization report they have no time to think—they are too busy producing results. Short-range thinking is symptomatic.

        Our experience of start-up is that during the first twelve to fifteen months the members of the organization work with a fanatical zeal. Their work day is twelve to fifteen hours long, and they spend six or seven days each week at the organization to get things done. While there may be many organizational policies and procedures on paper, they have not yet been integrated into behaviors. It is an exciting and draining time. The dysfunction during this time is known as "infant mortality." Perhaps because of a shortage of capital, the "infant" does not make it.
    3. Go-go. During the go-go time everything looks like an opportunity. There is a lot of E once more. Decisions are made intuitively, and the interest span is short.

We have experienced this in numerous departments marketing products to external audiences before the products were fully developed. The energy was to market every new form, software program, and so on that was developed. During this time in the organization's life cycle, the founder of the organization may be left behind. The organization may begin to take on its own life. There may be conflicts to be worked out as the original founder and the new members of the organization have differences of opinion. The dysfunction at this stage is the "founder" or "family trap."
4. Adolescence. Adolescence is a time of increasing the A. The organization is settling in. There are more policies and procedures coming into place. Decisions are made by a defined process instead of impulsively. Planning takes on a new dimension. In discussions the question will be asked: How does this fit with our plan? The dysfunction is that the organization stays locked into trying to be entrepreneurial and does not focus. The result can be a splinter group (divorce) or premature aging of the organization.
5. Prime. The organization in its prime is running at maximum. There is a strong combination of the P, A, I, and a planned E function. The organization is energetic and predictable. It knows what it can and cannot achieve. The goal for organizations is to remain in the prime. One key is to keep the E function going.
6. Stable. The stable organization drops some of the E focus and focuses the energy on results, policies, and integration. The climate is formal, and new ideas are not received with excitement.

B. Descending curve
1. Aristocracy. In the first aristocracy, the climate is stale. Everything is okay as long as no waves are made. People are nice, and it is important to be polite. However, there is an eroding of market share, and the P side of the organization may begin to drop off.
2. Early bureaucracy. This phase is one with a clear de-

Understanding the Culture of the Organization

cline of P. There may be some open fighting between managers. Someone may have to take the "fall," that is, the organization may be looking for scapegoats. The A function is strong, and much of the rest of the functions are weak.

3. Bureaucracy. The A energies are clear here. The key focus will be on the written word with much agreement but not much accomplishment. It will not be unusual to think we have come to an understanding but to have no action grow out of it.

    If you work with this type of organization, you may find that you need to create a bypass mechanism. For example, in working with government bureaucracy you may need to create a legislative lobby.

4. Death. Eventually the organization dies. A fact of all life is that birth begets death. Death for an organization might be going out of business or merging with another business.

The above is one model of the stages of an organization's life cycle. We believe that it is very useful for the internal consultant to have a sense of the stage of development of the organization or the department in which he or she is working.

In the early life of the organization, the internal consultant's role is to help establish boundaries. Typically, there is a good deal of energy and excitement, and the role is one of directing and managing that energy. The consultant helps provide a focus and helps select from the many options.

On the descending side of the curve the consultant's role is to unfreeze. Typically the organization has locked into its culture and needs to be broken free. This means confronting the current situation and helping to create options.

The assessment questions for the internal consultant are:

1. How much focus does this organization have on producing an effective product?
2. How much entrepreneurial spirit is there? When was the last new idea or product produced?

3. How much of the work is predefined by policies and procedures? Are they locked in?
4. How well are things integrated?
5. Do I need to help divert energy or confront staleness?

Summary

This chapter has been about the organizational culture in which the internal consultant works. The internal consultant must learn to be sensitive to the culture in which he or she is. Culture sets the parameters of what can be done and how it can be done. Culture defines the norms out of which people will relate to each other, and those norms impact how the internal consultant will chart his or her work.

We also discussed the concept of organizational life cycles. We believe that organizations are constantly unfolding, and it is imperative for the internal consultant to be aware of this.

The bottom line of this chapter is this: consultations do not happen in a vacuum. They happen in an organizational culture. That means the internal consultant needs to take a broader perspective than simply viewing the immediate intervention. The consultant needs to be sensitive to the organizational ramifications of her or his work.

9

Sharpening Four Essential Interpersonal Skills

We have discussed the role of the internal consultant, the process of internal consulting, and the environment of the internal consultant. With each step of the internal consulting process we included a skills checklist for that stage of the consulting process. However, there are some general skills that are necessary throughout the internal consulting process. These skills have to do with listening, influence, conflict management, and problem solving. This chapter will discuss listening skills, influence skills, conflict management skills, and problem-solving skills.

Interpersonal Skills

Listening skills are vital for the internal consultant. Without them the whole consulting process comes to a halt. Again, let us return to the basic foundation of the helpee and helper. The only way the helper can be helpful is to first understand the nature of the other person's problem. It is a matter of listening to the thoughts and feelings of the client.

Influencing skills are the second set of skills needed. A key part of the internal consultant role is influencing the other person. Our definition of the role of internal consultant is built on the foundation of a helper-helpee relationship. It is a reality that influence skills are critical for the internal consultant. Our approach will be to look at influence from power bases — what are the power bases from which the internal consultant can work?

Third, we consider skills in the management of conflict. Throughout the internal consulting process, conflict will be a reality. Remember the discussion of the pinch model? Pinches will happen. That means that the internal consultant needs a good command of conflict management skills. We will provide some suggestions for the management of conflict in the consulting process.

Fourth, we present ideas on problem solving. As stated earlier, the work of the internal consultant is primarily that of a problem solver. That is why he or she is requested to come into an organization. We will provide two very specific processes for use.

The process of skill building for the internal consultant never stops. It is not something that one stops doing. It is truly lifelong learning.

Listening Skills: The Way into the Other's World

Countless books and articles have been written about listening skills. Listening is one of the major skills that the internal consultant needs. This means listening to the client's perception of the problems and what got them to where they are. This means listening to the client's feelings, which are background to the problem. It means listening to the data that are collected. It means listening to the responses to the data when they are presented. And, finally, it means listening to the evaluation of the consult.

Obviously we are talking about more than just the physical skill of listening. We are talking about the ability to let a problem talk to you. Ulschak (1978, pp. 148–153) represents part of our view in his discussion of systems analysis as a tool for letting the problem talk to you. The key is being open and receptive to what the client and the problem are saying to you.

Listening skills refers here to what is said and how it is said. Both the verbal and the nonverbal are critical elements in

Sharpening Four Essential Interpersonal Skills 195

the communication. The classic verbal-nonverbal illustration is of the person who is leaning back in a chair with her arms folded across her chest saying, "I am really open to what you are saying..." The verbal is saying one thing, and the nonverbal is saying something else.

Here are two exercises that will focus the verbal and the nonverbal.

Verbal. Sit down with another person at least once a day and practice listening skills. Practice by reflecting back to the other person what you are hearing from him. Start by reflecting the words: "What I hear you saying is..." Let him know that you in fact are listening.

Then move to reflecting the feelings that you are sensing. Phrases such as "What I hear you saying is... and I sense that you are feeling... Is that correct?"

The whole purpose of the exercise is to get inside the other person and understand what his world is like. You are to move out of you and into his world.

Practice this once a day for thirty days, and your listening skills will be greatly enhanced.

Nonverbal. Once a day for the next thirty days, simply observe the nonverbal behaviors of those around you. Do not judge or arrive at conclusions. Simply observe. Pick a specific person and simply observe. How does she walk? How does she use or not use her hands when she is speaking? What about her eyes? Does she make eye contact or not?

The goal is to simply observe. Again, by getting into a habit of observing behaviors, you will increase your own awareness of the other person and his or her world.

The two exercises are useful in expanding your awareness with regard to listening. However, even more important than the techniques of listening is the desire to understand. We have all had the privilege of being in the presence of a person who has learned the "listening technique." We know that because every time we say something, that person responds with, "What I hear you saying is . . ." We get tired of the response after a while if we sense that the person is really not listening but simply using a technique. The technique is an aid and not the end.

We need to come into the setting with the client with one objective—to understand as fully as possible that person's world of behaviors, thoughts, and feelings.

We are really talking here about an attitude toward the client that invites the client to disclose his or her world to us. The technique is simple, but the attitude can be difficult. Here are some hints to enhance your listening skills:

1. Be sure to have your meeting in an environment that is conducive to listening.
2. Establish as a goal for the meeting that you want to understand the other person's world.
3. As the person talks, reflect back to her or him what you have heard and ask for confirmation, for example, "What I hear you saying is . . . Is that correct?"
4. Remember, listen not only for the words but for the feelings of the person as well.
5. Finish the meeting by asking, "What have I not heard that I need to hear?"

Influence Skills

Influence skills are vital for the internal consultant. The consultant starts by trying to understand how he or she goes about influencing others. What are the ways the consultant goes about influencing the client? Remember, typically the internal consultant is not in a position of authority over the client. Any influencing that is done is done in other ways.

It is necessary that the internal consultant have self-awareness of how he or she goes about the influence process. Remember the Johari window that we discussed in Chapter Two? It is a useful tool for increasing your self-awareness regarding influence skills.

Take a moment and evaluate your influence skills by thinking about the following questions. Think back to a recent

Sharpening Four Essential Interpersonal Skills 197

time when you wanted to influence a decision maker in your life. How did you influence this person? What specifically did you do? What was the response? When you were done, what was your feeling? Were you successful?

Pay attention to several things in your answers. First, did you actually develop strategies ahead of time about the person and the best way to approach him or her? This is frequently a weak area with internal consultants. Internal consultants need to take time to think about the client and his or her needs or wants and then decide the best strategy for approaching the client.

Second, what did you feel when you were done? This is an important piece of data concerning your level of comfort with influencing another person. Do you feel successful?

Third, and most important, did you get done what needed to get done? This is the results question: "When all is said and done, did you get what was needed?"

One of the most important understandings that the consultant needs to have in mind is what he or she wants. The consultant needs to think, "What do I want from this person?" and "What do I think this person wants from me?" These questions are clarifiers—they assist the consultant in clarifying her or his own agenda for the meeting.

There are many ways to approach influencing skills. We will approach influencing skills here through power bases. In the next few pages we will discuss the internal consultant role from the viewpoint of power bases. Then we will invite you to think about your use of these power bases.

Hersey and Natemeyer (1979) have identified seven power bases that are useful for us to consider in the context of the internal consultant. These are:

1. *Coercive power.* Coercive power is based on the ability to punish. If you can create fear in the other person, you have coercive power. If you work with coercive power, people will respond to you because they perceive that you have the ability to punish them.

2. *Connectional power.* This is based on the internal consultant's connections with other people in the organization. While

most internal consultants do not have coercive power, many have connectional power. They know important people in the organization. People respond to the internal consultant because they perceive he or she has influence on other influential people.

3. *Expert power*. Expert power comes from being seen as an expert in an area. The internal consultant has this power because he knows how things are done.

4. *Informational power*. Informational power has to do with the internal consultant's perceived ability to get certain kinds of information. An analogy might be the secretary who has power because she knows what goes on in a board meeting. The internal consultant may not be an expert, but he knows how to get the information and has an inside track to it.

5. *Legitimate power*. Legitimate power is the power that a person gets because of her position in the organization. Others will respond to her because they perceive that she is in a position of authority. This person is a manager or administrator.

6. *Referent power*. Referent power is the power that comes with personality. The internal consultant has a dynamic personality that inspires people to respond to him. He has charisma.

7. *Reward power*. Reward power is the ability to reward persons. Others listen because they believe that the internal consultant has the power of reward.

Note that in all of these it is other persons' perceptions that are critical. It is other persons' perception that the consultant can reward them that causes them to respond. It is other persons' perception that the consultant has the expert information that causes them to respond. This is a vital learning for the internal consultant—your power rests in other persons' perceptions of you. This means that those other persons give us our influence.

Take a moment and think back to those seven power bases. Which of those is your strongest? Which is your second strongest? When you think back to a time when you wanted to influence a decision maker, from what power base did you come? Which of the power bases do you normally not use? Which are the ones that you avoid? How does that limit you?

Sharpening Four Essential Interpersonal Skills

Figure 21. Power Base Assessment.

Power Base	+	0	−
1. Coercive			
2. Connectional			
3. Expert			
4. Informational			
5. Legitimate			

Take a moment and do the following exercise using the chart in Figure 21. Rate yourself on your use of each power base. If it is one that you are familiar with and that you use frequently, give it a +. If it is one that you think you use some, give it a 0. If it is one that you never use, give it a −.

The major power bases for most internal consultants are expert power, information power, referent power, and connection power. Typically, the internal consultant does not have the power to reward or punish, only the power to provide information, connect with others, and be an expert.

Here are examples of the use of each of these four power bases:

1. *Expert power.* The human resource office is advising a department on the process of disciplinary action. The manager has been lax in documenting an employee's performance, and human resources is providing expertise in the disciplinary process and its implications.

2. *Information power.* The internal consultant is gathering information on retention for a nursing department. The information relates to the creative responses that can be found in the literature.

3. *Referent power.* The internal consultant uses her personal charisma to get approval of a project that reviews the exit interviews. Normally, she would not be able to access those records, but because of her personal presentation, she is able to do so.

4. *Connectional power.* This is major for internal consultants, who typically are well connected in the organization. They

travel around to different parts of the organization and know what is going on. This means that they have a certain degree of power because of their connections.

A specific example is the consultant who is doing a turnover study in a department. The consultant is there because the department manager's boss has requested the study. This means that the consultant has a special connectional link to the manager's boss, with some associated power.

The internal consultant has the ability to reward and punish only indirectly. For example, we have a client who calls us in annually to do some work. The work is typically meaningful and worthy. However, the time also coincides with the client's performance review. He works for someone who rewards being proactive, and his using our consulting service is seen as being proactive. The manager is rewarded because he uses us. This means that indirectly we have a reward ability.

In another department the reverse is true. We are there at the request of the manager, but the work has potentially damaging implications for the manager. The result of our intervention in the department might well be a "punishment" for the manager.

We have introduced the concepts. Take a few moments and think about how you use power bases to influence those around you. You may even want to talk to a few of them about how they see you influencing them.

Again, we encourage you to take some time and think about your strong power bases and how they are useful for you and your weak power bases and how they limit you. You might take some time and talk with some former clients about your learnings. How do your former clients perceive you?

Some of you may be asking: But how does this relate to influence styles? Simply put, the power bases that I use are my influence strategies. By learning from which bases I work, I can expand my ability to influence by increasing my options. For example, it is not unusual to find an internal consultant who has strong expert power but does not recognize his or her referent or connectional power. These become "blind spots." By taking time

Sharpening Four Essential Interpersonal Skills

to work with the power bases, he or she can begin to increase influence skills.

It is humbling to revisit power bases. Why? Because power bases are in the eyes of the beholder. It is the other person who allows us to use a power base. We only can influence the other person when that person lets us. That person is the doorkeeper. This means that we once again need to talk with others about how they see us. We can say, "Here are the power bases out of which I work." However, the other person is really the one to say, "Here is why I respond to you." We can speculate about our power bases—others know how it is they let us influence them.

The CPR + F model is an excellent framework from which to approach influence. Prior to a meeting with an individual you want to influence, think through the following questions:

1. What is my purpose in this meeting? What do I want from this other person? What does that person want from me? What am I willing to give up to achieve my want, and what is the other person willing to give up? Key to any influence strategy is knowing what you want from the other person and your boundaries for that want.

2. How committed am I to that want? If 10 on a ten-point scale means I am highly committed to it, am I a 3 or a 7? This focuses the question of how invested you are to the want. Take time to ask yourself: How important is this for me? How much do I have invested in it? What role does the other person want to have in the meeting?

3. What role do I want to take in the meeting? Do I want to be a director and set the agenda? Do I simply want to be the facilitator and work from that framework? What role do I want?

4. What will be my clues in the meeting that say I am on track with purpose and roles? How will I know if I have a shift in commitment? Feedback is vital throughout the meeting to see that I remain on target. It provides the "score."

Figure 22 summarizes the CPR + F approach to influence.

Being influenced and influencing are vital to the consulting relationship. Influencing will happen whether the consul-

Figure 22. CPR + F Applied to Influence.

	Other Person	Me
What is wanted from the meeting?		
How invested in the want?		
What role do I take in the meeting?		
Feedback—what are the clues?		

tant is aware of it or not. We believe that the consultant must be very intentional in influencing and being influenced.

Conflict Management Skills

The internal consultant also needs to have conflict management skills. Throughout the consultation process, it is a given that there will be conflict.

The question is not whether or not there will be conflict but how the conflict will be managed. In fact, if the internal consultant does not experience conflict, something is probably wrong, and he or she needs to seriously evaluate this.

We have several fundamental beliefs about conflict. First, conflict is a given condition of life. Think about a typical day at work. There are conflicts about work priorities. There are conflicts because people do things in a way that others do not like. There are conflicts about the amount of time a person spends at work and at home.

Second, conflict is a source of energy. Conflict is an energizer for new thoughts and creativity. If you think that strange, the next time you are bored go out and pick a fight—you will be energized quickly. The important point is that conflict is an

Sharpening Four Essential Interpersonal Skills 203

energy source that can be most useful for an individual or organization when effectively utilized.

Third, conflict is a time of creative birthing of something new. Out of conflict comes a new potential. Think of conflicts of which you have been part where the outcome has been something creative. Properly handled conflict has rich potential for creating new ideas and approaches to problems.

Fourth, an individual's response to a conflict setting is built on what she or he has learned about conflict in the past. Again, we are back to the percept model. If we have learned that conflict is negative and destructive, we will want to avoid conflict when we experience it. However, if in the past we have learned that conflict is a natural part of life and we can learn from it, we will treat conflict as an opportunity when it arises.

We often use the metaphor of the thunderstorm in our work with individuals and departments in the management of conflict. Thunderstorms represent the conflict cycle. Think about the last time that you experienced a thunderstorm. First, the storm appears on the horizon. There are the changes in temperature. Perhaps the wind comes up. There is a sense of the storm's coming, but there is a possibility that it might pass over. Then the storm is upon you. There are thunder, lightning, and the downpour of rain. The sky is dark and forbidding. It can be a scary time—a time to go down to the basement and hide. Then, at some point, the storm begins to recede. The wind is not as harsh and the rain not as heavy. Maybe sunlight breaks through the clouds. Gradually, the clouds pass over you. The other side of the storm is refreshment. The air is fresh. The earth has been watered once more. There may or may not be some destruction in the storm's path—but there is a newness with its passing.

The conflict cycle is like that thunderstorm. It starts with some storm clouds on the horizon. Think about the last conflict you were in. Rarely are there not some clouds on the horizon that say a conflict is around. Conflicts are a constant part of the health care scene. There are conflicts of purpose, role, and commitment. There are conflicts of structural differences. The point—there are constantly conflicts waiting to materialize.

Then the storm builds, and the conflict is full blown. In

the conflict cycle model we say that is the time when we become aware that a storm is brewing. We perceive there is a conflict. Once we perceive the conflict, we move to our behaviors and attitudes about conflict. For some that means confronting the conflict; for others, avoiding it. For still others that means waiting it out. Whatever our response, we move from a time of perception to a time of acting on the perception. This is the key area for managing the conflict. Our behaviors at this point can exacerbate or diminish the conflict.

Gradually, the conflict works itself over, and the sun comes through on the other side. Most conflicts, if allowed to move through the cycle, have on their other side a refreshing newness. The problem with conflict management happens when we cut the conflict management cycle short and do not learn from the conflict. In such a case there is a tendency to sweep things under the rug and begin to build for a new conflict. Referring back to the pinch model, we are storing stamps.

Some of the positive results of living through the conflict include:

- reaffirmation of purpose, roles, and commitment
- definition of the issues involved
- identification of dissent and dissatisfaction
- stimulation of the search for new facts and solutions
- prevention of stagnation
- formation of group cohesion

Some of the negative results of not living through the conflict include:

- increase of bitterness
- disruption of work setting
- disagreements going underground
- lack of role agreement and clarity
- increased work tension and stress

Most of the time we can feel if we are closing the conflict too soon. The important point is that conflict is a cycle that is

Sharpening Four Essential Interpersonal Skills

Figure 23. Conflict Management Cycle.

```
┌─────────────┐                          ┌─────────────┐
│ Milieu of   │─────────────────────────▶│ Perception  │
│ potential   │                          │ of conflict:│
│ conflicts   │      Awakening           │ threshold of│
└─────────────┘         to               │ awareness   │
                      conflict           └─────────────┘
       ┌──────────────┐                         │
       │ Aftermath:   │                         ▼
       │ residue contro│                 ┌─────────────┐
       │ or resolution │                 │ Mulling:    │
       └──────────────┘                  │ finding     │
              ▲                          │ out more    │
              │                          │ about       │
              │                          └─────────────┘
              │    ┌──────────┐                ▲
              └────│ Action/  │────────────────┘
                   │ responses│
                   └──────────┘
```

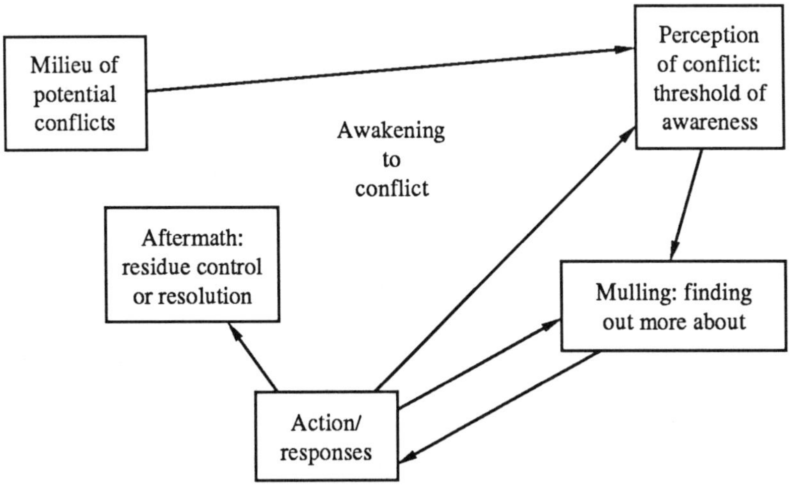

lived through, good things can come out of conflict, and on the other side of the storm is the freshness of new possibilities.

That is essentially what the conflict cycle is all about. The problem is that we sometimes get stuck in the storm and do not let the cycle take its natural course. We need to find ways to let the conflict cycle work itself through. Conflict is an important friend of the internal consultant, and when we own that conflict as a friend, we are on the right track to effective conflict management.

The analogy of a fever is appropriate here. When the thermometer says one hundred degrees, we tend not to avoid it but rather begin to respond to it. The fever is a sign that something is not right. Conflict is another sign that something is not right. Maybe my expectations are not in line with yours. Maybe we have different goals or ways of doing things. The conflict simply reveals that something here needs attention.

The conflict management cycle is illustrated in Figure 23.

What needs to happen in settings where conflict is likely? We distinguish two general types of settings. The first setting is when you anticipate the conflict, and the purpose of the setting is to get the conflict out. Conflict is anticipated and even planned for. The second is when the conflict comes unexpectedly. As we say in the business, you get "blind-sided."

In the planned setting, there are a number of things to be done. First of all, take time *prior* to the session to work with the others involved to:

1. Clarify the purpose of the meeting. Remember, the meeting is not to "get" a person. It is to resolve a problem. That is the focus. Work with the other members of the meeting so there is a common agreement on the purpose and focus of the meeting. Our experience is that differences of purpose are one of the four most common sources of conflict.

2. Clarify the roles of the persons involved in the meeting. No one should turn up at the meeting without knowing the roles of the individuals. Role conflict and the lack of role clarity are the second most common sources of conflicts. When people do not understand or agree with their roles or the roles of others, there will be conflict.

3. Clarify the level of commitment the parties need to resolve the conflict. This is the third most common source of conflict. In any significant issue there will be different levels of commitment to the resolution of conflicts. Some individuals will have high levels of commitment, and others will not. Some may actually enjoy the conflict and find it a source of personal power. As long as everyone is focused on the conflict, no one is looking at what might be the real issue. We sometimes look too much at the fire and not enough at what is happening around the fire.

4. Clarify the feedback mechanism and channels. This is the fourth most common area of organizational conflict. People do not have good information regarding what is going on and how it is happening. They need feedback channels.

5. Clarify others' perceptions of the problems. If the meeting is problem oriented, take time to understand what others see as the problem. This may be done through the use of questionnaires or interviews. Perhaps part of the meeting could be a time of problem clarification. Having the participants share what they see as the conflict and the sources of the conflict in the meeting can be very useful.

This is all presession work with the others involved. In

Sharpening Four Essential Interpersonal Skills

addition, plan when and where you want the meeting to happen. For example, you probably do not want it in the middle of the cafeteria. Structure the meeting so that successful resolution of the conflict is probable.

Some hints for the meeting setting include:

1. Be sensitive to confidentiality — select a room that provides for confidentiality.
2. Try to select a room that is neutral ground for the parties involved.
3. Make sure that sufficient time is allocated for the meeting.
4. Have the room set up so that all of the participants can readily see one another.
5. Monitor beepers and other paging devices. Ideally, have beepers checked at the door. There is nothing quite so distracting as a beeper's going off and people's moving around.

In the actual meeting, it is important to review the purpose of and to develop ground rules for the meeting. We like to do this by asking the participants how they would like to live out the next hour. What environment would they like to create to facilitate the problem solving? What behaviors do we need to have? What behaviors would they not want to have?

The important point is this — if you know there is going to be conflict, set up the meeting in such a way that the conflict is effectively managed. Conflict meetings can be fun and stimulating because of the energy of conflict. The key is managing that energy.

The second setting is when you have unexpected conflict. For the first few minutes you may be knocked off balance by the conflict, and that is okay. If the conflict is intense, it may take more than a few minutes for you to get back on your feet. Remember, when we perceive conflict, our body has a physical response to fight or flee. When that fight or flight response happens, our body begins to pour stored sugar and fats into the bloodstream, increase the breathing rate, speed up the heart, cease digestion, and so on. The body is physically responding to the signal we have given it that a conflict is present. If you are caught off guard by conflict, expect that before your conscious mind knows it, your body will be preparing for the fight or flight. The sayings to "count to ten" or "take a break" or "bite your tongue" all have at their core a distancing from the immediate fight or flight response. Then you regain your composure, and the body can return to normal.

The first task, then, is to give yourself some "breathing room." With a minor conflict this might be a minute or so to regroup. Take a few deep breaths and concentrate on your breathing. With a a major conflict this might mean taking a break from the meeting. The goal is to give yourself time after your immediate reaction to the conflict. Once you have recovered from the initial reaction, the second task is to move to active listening. Active listening means that you actively try to understand the other person's point of view. By moving to active listening, you switch from a fight or flight mode to an understanding mode. It is not unusual to have two or more parties in the disagreement suddenly realize that they are saying the same thing—there really is not a conflict. So, the second task is to recover from the immediate response and say, "Help me understand what you are saying."

The third task is to hear fully what the person is saying and then state your position. Again, the discipline of active listening can keep you engaged in a way that lets you assess what the issue is. During the listening you may have discovered one of the following:

- There is no issue but simply a misunderstanding.
- There is a clear difference of opinion with regard to purpose, role, or commitment.
- The problem is still messy and unclear.

The fourth task is to state what you feel and think regarding the issue and to invite the others to hear you fully.

Now that the conflict is on the table, it is time to begin to explore alternative responses. This is the fifth task. Generally, in any conflict setting, there are four options:

Sharpening Four Essential Interpersonal Skills 209

1. *Ignore or avoid the conflict.* As you are well aware, many conflicts are best ignored. They are minimal, and focusing on them would be a waste of resources. At other times the conflict is "hot," and you may want to ignore it for a while so it can cool down.

2. *Confront the conflict head on.* This is the aggressive/assertive approach. It takes the bull by the horns. It is surgical—if the issue centers on a person, remove the person.

But it is more than this. It is simply walking into someone's office and saying, "I think we have a conflict here, and I would like to discuss it." That is straightforward and direct without being aggressive. This approach means stating what the wants are and where the conflict resides.

3. *Work at compromises to the conflict.* Compromise means that each of the parties involved will lose something. I know what I want, and I know what I am willing to accept. You know what you want, and you know what you are willing to accept. Each of us will lose a bit of what we want for what we can get. The goal is to have the mutual losses be minor.

4. *Create a new something.* This is the exciting option. It is the one that results in a creative birthing from the conflict.

The sixth task is to act and then evaluate. You have heard the other person, you have explained your options. Now it is time to act and then evaluate to see if the conflict has been managed or controlled.

Following are some specific ways to address conflict in one-on-one encounters and in groups:

1. Ahead of time, identify your wants in the relationship and what you are willing to negotiate for those wants.
2. Role-play through the conflict with another person. If you are not comfortable with that, role-play in front of a mirror where you can visualize yourself in the setting.
3. Identify the worst possible outcomes of this conflict. Then note them. How probable are they?
4. Plan for damage control. If everything were to "blow up," how would you manage the damage?

5. Decide if the best strategy is to confront the conflict, let it be, or ignore it.
6. Identify what part of the conflict is your responsibility. Know what part of it you own.
7. Take time to plan out when and how the conflict will be discussed. Also, plan the setting in which the conflict session will take place.
8. Be careful to not define the problem as a person—personality conflicts define problems in a "non-problem-solving" frame. Define the problem in terms of behaviors.

Conflict is a given. The task for the internal consultant is to turn the conflict into something positive.

Problem Solving

The major work of the internal consultant is that of problem solver. Problems are what cause the internal consultant to be invited in to work. If the client did not have a problem or a potential problem, he or she would not have contacted the internal consultant. The internal consultant's role is to work with the client in resolving current problems or preventing future problems.

Three Types of Problems

Problems represent some type of deviation from the expected. Things were going along fine, and then there was a deviation. Now we have a problem. There is a gap between what is desired and what is.

We have three descriptions of approaching problems as gaps between what is and what is desired. They are represented in the model shown in Figure 24.

Type 1 Problems: Identifying What Is. The first type of problem deals with identification of what is. We are interested in identifying the current conditions that are creating the perception that a problem exists.

Figure 24. Problem Solving: Moving from What Is to the Desired.

(Movement from A to B)

```
A ─────────────────────▶ B
Current (what is)        Desired
```

This is the part of the process that focuses on *what is*. "Describe the current conditions." "Identify changes that have been made recently that may contribute to the problem's becoming a problem." The focus is on the current conditions causing the problem and keeping the problem from resolving itself.

Type 2 Problems: Knowing the Desired State. This is a problem of knowing what is desired. Where is it that we would like to go? Is this the desired state that we want?

The focus here is not on the current condition but on the desired condition. This means taking time to identify what the conditions would be if there were no problem.

Typically, we ask questions like, "If this problem were resolved, what would we be hearing and seeing? What would be happening differently?" Again, we describe that desired future as specifically as possible.

Type 3 Problems: Selecting Alternatives. This is the problem of what alternative to select to get from A to B. Some alternatives are productive and will quickly resolve the problem. Others are not. The goal is to identify the most effective alternative.

The key here is making a decision regarding alternatives. It becomes a decision-making process.

All three types of problems will arise in the work of the internal consultant. There are unique questions to be asked for each problem type. Each of these problem types has a different set of accompanying questions. Here are some examples:

Type 1 problems: identifying what is
When did the problem begin?
Who was involved with the problem?
When was it first identified? By whom? How?

What changes occurred just prior to the problem's appearing in the problem environment?
    People changes?
    Technology changes?
    Environmental changes?
Is there a probable cause of the problem? If so, what is it?
    How certain are we that it is the probable cause?
Does the probable cause explain the above?

Type 2 problems: identifying the desired state
Who needs to be involved in identifying the desired state?
Who has vested interests?
What is the desired future?
    People?
    Technology?
    Other
What would indicate that the desired is happening?
How is that desired state different from the current state?

Type 3 problems: selecting alternatives
Who needs to be involved in the selection of alternatives?
    Who has information for us that will be useful in our determining alternatives?
What is the cost benefit of the alternatives? Are some choices obviously much better than others?
What is the most effective alternative?
What is the most efficient alternative?

    We can talk about a problem as being a problem for which we do not know the present conditions, desired future states, or alternatives for moving from the present to the future. We may know the desired state but not the current state. In other words, it is a problem of determining the causes of the problem. We can also have problems for which we know the current causes but not the desired future. There are also problems for which we know both the causes and the desired future but not the best alternative for getting from the present to that future. For example, we are in the process of getting a new computer system. We know the cause of the current problems, and we know the

Sharpening Four Essential Interpersonal Skills 213

desired future. Now we are in the process of making the decision regarding the best alternatives for getting from the present to the future.

Finally, there are problems that involve all three—the causation is unknown, the future is unknown, and the alternatives are hazy. This is known as a "mess." A friend of mine likes to use the analogy of fishing to describe this type of problem.

If you have ever gone fishing with worms, you have probably had the experience of the worms' grouping together in the bottom of the can and getting totally entwined. As a result, it is almost impossible to get a single worm from the can. You simply grab one worm and work on it until it finally comes out and continue this process until the worms are untangled.

Most really good problems are messy problems. They do not have easy, obvious solutions. The only approach is to start somewhere—grab one of the worms and pull until that problem becomes clear, and then move on to the next problem. These messy problems have confusion in two or more of the problem types.

We will provide specific suggestions in the next section of this chapter.

Problem-Solving Process

There are many processes available for problem solving. Ulschak, Nathanson, and Gillan (1981) provide a good resource for a number of the processes available. The processes are useful for individuals or groups in approaching problem solving.

What is a problem-solving process? Essentially, a problem-solving process is a logical, step-by-step approach to thinking through a problem. Some processes are very specific to current conditions, others are focused on determining future conditions, and still others are decision-making processes for deciding how to move from the present to the future.

An overview of generic problem-solving steps is found in Ulschak, Nathanson, and Gillan (1981, p. 2). The steps are:

1. *Awareness of problem.* The start of the problem-solving process is the recognition that something is not quite right. There is a gap between what is and what is desired.
2. *Problem diagnosis and identification.* This is a time of determining exactly what the problem is. Again, the assumption is that most problem solving starts with a presenting problem that may or may not be the central problem.
3. *Selection of criteria for solution.* How will you know if the problem has been solved? For many of us in the midst of problem solving, this sounds simplistic. However, it is important to specify what the solution will look like.
4. *Formulation of alternatives.* Once the diagnosis and the criteria are established, the next step is to formulate possible strategies for resolving the problem.
5. *Selection of strategy.* Now we select which strategy is best. This means looking at the criteria for solution and saying, "Which of these strategies is most effective in getting those criteria met?"
6. *Specification of action plan.* Now is the time to turn the strategy into an action plan with specifics to implement the strategy.
7. *Implementation of action plan.* The plan has been developed, and now it is implemented.
8. *Monitoring and evaluation.* Did the problem get corrected? Was the action plan carried out? This is a time of review.

The above is a generic model for thinking through a problem. Each of the steps has specific subquestions. However, we present it here as a general framework for problem solving.

Most processes will have two central parts. The first part is the expanding of immediate options. This is the *expansion phase*. Frequently, it is referred to as "brainstorming." The goal is to develop a multitude of options. Possible questions are: What are the causes of this problem? What are the solutions to this problem? What is the best way to address this problem?

The questions should be worded in such a way that they invite alternatives. Generally, there is a ground rule preventing evaluation of ideas at this time. The goal is to expand the options.

Sharpening Four Essential Interpersonal Skills

Figure 25. Brainstorming How Tos.

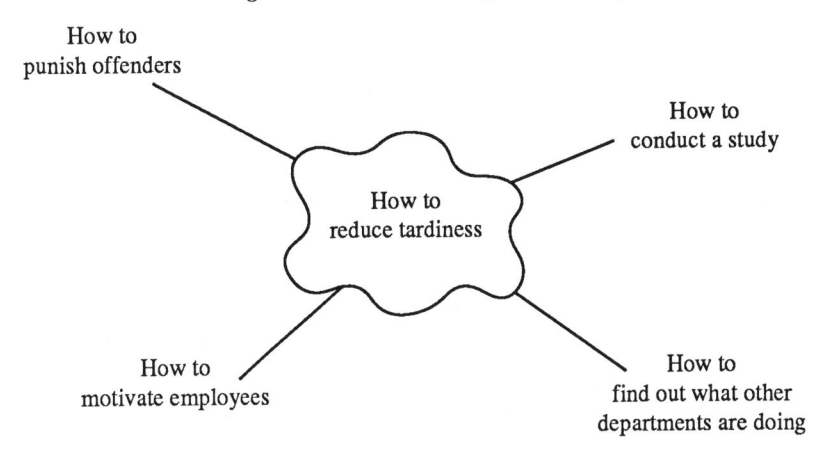

- How to punish offenders
- How to conduct a study
- How to reduce tardiness
- How to motivate employees
- How to find out what other departments are doing

The *contraction phase* is the phase where the alternatives developed in the previous session are evaluated as possible solutions. We look at each alternative in light of the impact of that solution on the problem. Will this solution resolve the problem? What are the negative results of picking the solution? This is the evaluating phase of problem solving. Questions such as: Which of these are most feasible? and Which of these have the greatest probability for success? might be asked.

Here is a "quick and dirty" tool that is useful in thinking through a problem. It illustrates expansion and contraction. Simply follow these steps:

1. Write the problem about which you are thinking in the center of a sheet of paper. State the problem in a "how to" format. An example is:

How to reduce tardiness in my department

2. Now, brainstorm all your how tos. Write them on various places on the paper and connect them by a line to the problem statement (see Figure 25). Examples of other how tos are:

How to conduct a study on tardiness
How to find out what other departments are doing to address this issue
How to motivate employees to be here on time
How to hire self-responsible employees
How to punish offenders more effectively
How to deal more effectively with my frustration with this problem
How to determine if there is a pattern with tardiness

Note that every How to becomes a possible solution or a possible other problem to be addressed. Your feelings regarding this problem are also legitimate how tos. This is the expansion mode.

3. Now comes the contracting mode. This involves developing a set of criteria. It might mean that you rate each of the how tos developed on its potential as a solution. Will it resolve the problem in a timely way?

Most problem solving involves a period of time of expanding and contracting.

Problem-Solving Process: Two Examples

Earlier we suggested a generic model for problem solving. This section provides two problem-solving processes for your consideration. The goal is to present them in such a manner that you can readily use them. We provide a short walk-through with each method to illustrate it.

Force Field Analysis. Force field analysis comes from Kurt Lewin's (1935) effort to work with field theory to explain social changes. It is concerned with which forces keep the problem from being resolved and which forces move the problem toward resolution. The first are referred to as the *restraining forces*. They resist the solution of the problem. The second are the *facilitating forces*. They push the problem toward resolution.

Force field analysis involves identifying the restraining forces, the facilitating forces, the strength of each, and ways to

Sharpening Four Essential Interpersonal Skills 217

Figure 26. Force Field T Chart.

Restraining Forces	Facilitating Forces

reduce the restraining forces and increase the facilitating forces. We will take one step at a time.

First, with an individual or group, take time to define what the problem is. This is the start of any problem-solving process, but it is especially important in force field analysis. Second, identify the forces keeping the problem a problem and the forces trying to facilitate the resolution of the problem. We typically use the T chart shown in Figure 26.

Third, weight the forces. Some restraining forces will be more powerful than others. Identify the ones that are most crucial in restraining the problem. Then identify the forces that are moving the problem toward resolution. Which of these are strong? Which are crucial for problem resolution? A general principle with force field analysis is that it is better to remove or reduce restraining forces than to add facilitating forces because generally an increase in facilitating forces also adds new restraining forces.

Fourth, decide which restraining forces to reduce and which facilitating forces to strengthen. This is the action planning and strategy. The ideal is to remove the restraining forces and simply let the problem move to resolution. A specific action can be identified to reduce the effectiveness of each restraining force. A specific action can be developed to enhance each facilitating force.

Here is a brief walk-through of the process in action:

Problem: Low turnout at community education classes that health care institution is running.

Restraining forces: (forces keeping the problem a problem)
lack of advertising
lack of effective use of physicians' contacts

poor facilities
lack of needs assessment to see what community wants

After spending some time discussing these restraining forces, they were rank ordered as follows:
lack of needs assessment
lack of advertising
poor facilities
lack of effective use of physicians

Facilitating forces (forces pushing the problem toward resolution)
top management interest in and commitment to programs
sufficient budget
excited and enthusiastic staff

A rank order of the facilitating forces produced the following list:
excited and enthusiastic staff
sufficient budget
top management interest

Action plan: A specific action step was devised for each of the key restraining and facilitating forces. Again, the goal was to reduce the restraining forces and increase the facilitating forces. The example "lack of needs assessment" was identified as a restraining action. The action plan now reads that "a needs assessment will be done by the education department by fall. It will be designed to identify specific health issues of the community."

Nominal Group. The nominal group process is one of the most useful tools with which we work. The process can readily be used in both one-on-one and small-group problem-solving sessions. The process produces two results. First, the ideas for possible solutions are identified; second, those ideas are ranked in terms of their potential as a solution.

The first step is an identification of the problem. The problem is defined on a flip chart or a piece of paper. The

Sharpening Four Essential Interpersonal Skills

participants are then asked to silently identify every solution they see to the problem.

There is a purpose for the silence. It means that each member of the group puts down what he or she sees as the possible solutions or responses to the problem. Because the participants write in silence, ideas are not being censored, and participants are not being influenced by other members of the group.

The second step is a "round robin." The leader asks each member of the group to give one idea that she or he has written. The leader writes the idea on a flip chart in front of the room. It is important that there is no discussion of the items during this step. Otherwise, participants can become defensive. The goal is to get the items listed. Members are instructed that if their idea is exactly like an idea already mentioned, they may pass over it. However, if their idea is somewhat different, they are encouraged to share it. This continues until no more ideas are generated.

When putting up ideas, one hint is to use letters of the alphabet to label them (A through Z and then AA through ZZ, and so on). This will make the next step easier.

The third step is discussion of the ideas for clarification. It is most useful to simply walk through the list from A to the last idea and ask for comments on each one. It is important to keep the process moving, or you will spend a good deal of time on this step. Walk through the list and ask for key comments—not debates. Also, be sensitive to members of the group who feel a need to defend their particular ideas. It is important to comment on ideas and not the person behind the idea. This time is for clarification of ideas.

This step may also be a time of joining or consolidating some items. The group may want to pull together a number of items that say the same thing. However, this must be done carefully so that the original ideas do not get lost.

The fourth step is ranking the items. The ranking process is straightforward. Each member of the group is asked to select the five or seven items that she or he believes have the greatest potential for being solutions. Five is used if there are fewer than twenty-five items, and seven is used if there are twenty-six or more. Each member of the group is given either five or seven three-by-five-inch cards. He or she is then asked to do the following for each card. In the upper left corner of the card, he or she writes the label of the item (for example, item C). In the middle of the card, he or she writes the idea. This provides a check to make sure that the wrong label is not written on the card. In the lower right corner he or she puts down the rank. With five cards the rank is from 1 to 5, with 5 being the most important and 1 the least important.

The members of the group do this individually and then give the cards to the facilitator. The facilitator scores the ranking and presents the final tallies.

The process is extremely effective in obtaining ideas from a group and arriving at a consensus on the solution having the greatest potentials. The following is an example using this method.

Problem statement. The group was brought together to work on the problem of how to increase communication between departments.

Silent idea generation. The first step was for the facilitator to explain the group's purpose and to present the steps of the nominal process. She then asked the members to write down their ideas on how to address the issue of communication. They were given ten minutes to generate the ideas silently.

Round robin:

Facilitator: You have all had an opportunity to write down your ideas. Now we will go around the room, and I would like each of you to give me the idea that you think has the most merit. As you hear others talk, if they have an idea similar to yours do not automatically take your idea off the list. Listen carefully to the idea. If it is exactly like yours, cross it off your list. If it has some uniqueness, put it up. Who would like to begin?

First member: I think we need to have interdepartmental meetings on a monthly basis.

Second member: My best idea is to have a job-share program

Sharpening Four Essential Interpersonal Skills

                where we would spend a small bit of time in other departments...

(The ideas go on until all members of the group have exhausted their ideas. The facilitator is writing each idea and putting a letter of the alphabet in front of each.)

Idea discussion:

Facilitator: Now that we have the ideas up, we will go back through them. Since we have twenty-eight ideas, we will have to keep the discussion of each brief. If you have a statement of support or a critique, state it, and then we will go on to the next item.

Member: I very much agree with the monthly meetings...

Ranking:

Facilitator: Now that we have commented on the ideas, the next step is to rank order them. Each of you has been given five three-by-five cards. Pick out the five best ideas that we have listed. Then, on each card, in the upper left corner write the letter of the idea and in the middle of the card write the idea itself. Take a few moments to do this....

                Now that you have the five ideas on the cards, in the lower right corner of the card give the ranking of that idea. The best idea give a 5, the second best a 4, and so on. When you get that done, we will take a short break while I summarize the rankings.

(The break is optional. We use it because it gives us time to write the ideas. Otherwise, we write the rankings on the flip chart. We simply write the ranking beside each item and then produce the total score.)

Final listing:

Facilitator: Based on your rankings and voting, the top three actions are...

(If there are ties, note that both are important. The goal is to identify ideas, not to become too rigorous with the cutoffs.)

Problem-Solving Pitfalls and Suggestions

We have presented two specific problem-solving processes. The purpose of a problem-solving process is to provide a structure for organizing the thinking of a group or individual with regard to the problem and possible solutions.

One strong suggestion is to make the group's work visual. A good method is to put it on a flip chart so that everyone can see the steps and where the process is going. This becomes extremely valuable.

Working with a group can be a delightful experience, or it can be frustrating. Here are some hints that will make it more delightful than frustrating:

1. *Set the stage for the group.* Before the group gathers, there should be a general understanding of the nature of the group, who is there and why they were selected, the duration of the session, expected outcomes, and roles for the time.

2. *Begin the session with a statement of purpose.* If the person responsible for calling the group together is different from the facilitator, the responsible person needs to talk about the purpose, expected outcomes, time duration, and what is expected of the participants.

3. *Talk through a plan of the session.* This means identifying the steps of the process and what roles mean. Crucial to the success of groups is that the group be very clear on purpose and roles.

4. *Take questions and comments from the group.* It is important to gauge the group's commitment to the process. The reason the group is gathered is that the decision maker believes that the group can flesh things out better than can an individual. That means that we want to have each individual invested in the group's process. If there are lots of comments about the group's being a waste of time, for example, the problem solving should be delayed until misgivings are addressed. The group needs to be present and committed to participation.

Sharpening Four Essential Interpersonal Skills

5. *Practice active listening and ask that the participants practice it.* The intent is to hear and understand others' ideas. Each idea is valuable, and the effort will be to get as much out of each idea as possible.

6. *Use all members of the group.* If someone is not contributing, ask the person what his or her thoughts are. Again, everyone's contribution is of value or they would not have been asked to be there.

7. *Regard conflicts or differences as assets to the group.* Value them and explore each difference fully. Do not jump to a premature agreement or gloss over an issue. If you do you will recycle it in the near future.

8. *Do not let one person dominate the group.* Remember that the purpose of a group is to use the full group. If one person dominates, that means others are not sharing ideas. Jones (1986, pp. 55–66) has a number of suggestions on how to control the person who dominates. For example, if you know the person will dominate, plan the meeting to minimize the domination. This may mean assigning the person to take notes. It may mean talking to the person about the dysfunctional behavior. It may mean talking about the behavior when it happens in the group. Jones provides many options.

9. *Keep the group informed of where you are in the process.* We like to have a "road map" for the session on a sheet of newsprint posted on the wall. We then refer to it as we proceed through the session.

10. *Provide recognition of ideas that emerge.* There is no such thing as a dumb idea. Even an idea that has low probability for results can be noted. Support shows the group that you are open to ideas.

11. *Do not let the generation of ideas and the evaluation of ideas mix.* Have a clear transition from idea generation to idea evaluation.

12. *As leader, do not compete with the group.* If you do, they will quickly turn against you or stop giving ideas. Competing means that you try to get the group to accept your ideas.

Other Problem-Solving Ideas. We have focused on formal problem-solving processes. However, there are a number of other useful methods that can be used in problem solving. These methods are somewhat unorthodox but useful. Here are a few ideas and thoughts.

1. *Use the notebook approach.* Identify a problem on which you are working. Each day of the week write down your thoughts regarding the problem. At the end of one or two weeks, review the ideas.

2. *Use a group notebook.* Use the same principle as in the first suggestion except this time have a group of people write down solutions to a problem. At the end of a week or two, have them turn in the listing.

3. *Form a problem-solving task force that meets once a month and takes on a particular problem and develops a list of suggestions for managing the problem.* This can be either a formal or an informal group.

4. *Make use of metaphors in the discussion of a problem.* For example, in our team-building work questions might be: If this team were a family, what kind of family would it be? Who would be the father? Who is the mother? and so on. Metaphors are powerful tools for thinking through problems.

5. *Look to examples of how other industries solve your issue.* For example, if you have problems with managing a flow of people through the outpatient clinic, talk to some other industries regarding how they manage issues. You may be surprised at the carryover.

There are many things that can be done with problem solving that invite creative and innovative solutions. Take time to work with these when you can.

Conclusion

This chapter has been about skills. We have talked about skills needed at various points in the consultant process as well as four sets of skills vital to all internal consulting—listening skills, influence skills, conflict management skills, and problem-solving skills.

Listening skills are vital for the internal consultant. Without good listening skills, the process breaks down and self-

Sharpening Four Essential Interpersonal Skills   225

destructs. The goal for the internal consultant is to understand the world of the client. That means that he or she needs good listening skills.

Internal consulting involves influencing and being influenced. The internal consultant wants to influence the client in a certain way and at the same time is influenced by the client. This means that the internal consultant needs to be very aware of her or his influencing skills.

All of internal consulting involves management of conflict. That is the essence of the consulting role. The internal consultant needs to be able to identify causes of conflicts, develop plans to manage and resolve conflicts, implement those plans, and evaluate the results of the corrective actions.

Exhibit 12 contains a complete skill checklist for internal consulting. We developed the model based on our own experience, the Consultation Skills Inventory (1976), and McLagan (1983). Take some time to use it and to develop next steps for your growth and development.

Exhibit 12. Skill Checklist for Internal Consulting.

The following is a listing of skills needed for internal consulting. For each skill, rate yourself as:
- (+) — You are well skilled and competent in this skill.
- (0) — You are okay in this skill.
- (−) — You feel yourself lacking in this skill.

General Consultation Skills
___ 1. Ability to listen to others
___ 2. Ability to ask direct probing questions
___ 3. Ability to listen to self and be aware of own feelings
___ 4. Ability to understand organization
___ 5. Ability to get industry-specific information
___ 6. Ability to think before reacting
___ 7. Ability to be comfortable with education and skill background
___ 8. Ability to understand why in a helping profession
___ 9. Ability to separate personal from professional issues
___ 10. Ability to build an atmosphere of trust and openness
___ 11. Ability not to be needed
___ 12. Ability to say no
___ 13. Ability to let go
___ 14. Ability to take risks
___ 15. Ability to ask for help
___ 16. Ability to be flexible

Precontracting and Contracting
___ 17. Ability to negotiate, that is, manage differences between you and others
___ 18. Ability to close a contract, that is, reach agreements
___ 19. Ability to manage conflict and anger addressed at you
___ 20. Ability to manage conflict and anger addressed at someone else
___ 21. Ability to offer suggestions in an appropriate way
___ 22. Ability to draw out others, that is, create a safe environment for them to share their ideas
___ 23. Ability to accept the client's definition of the problem and start from there
___ 24. Ability to help the client solve his or her own problems
___ 25. Ability to be honest to the client about what you can realistically deliver
___ 26. Ability to set realistic goals for the client and yourself
___ 27. Ability to help the client clarify the problem
___ 28. Ability to cost out projects in terms of resource consumptions
___ 29. Ability to logically think through the problem with the client
___ 30. Ability to offer your own ideas freely
___ 31. Ability to provide the client with feedback in such a manner that it is most often heard and understood
___ 32. Ability to work with others whom you do not necessarily like or appreciate
___ 33. Ability to be flexible in your consulting style to meet the client's needs

Data Collection and Analysis
___ 34. Ability to determine a plan of data collection, analysis, and presentation
___ 35. Ability to determine the data needed for a consultation

Sharpening Four Essential Interpersonal Skills

Exhibit 12. Skill Checklist for Internal Consulting, Cont'd.

___ 36. Ability to obtain data needed for a consultation
___ 37. Ability to design questions that get the needed information for questionnaires and interviews
___ 38. Ability to use library resources in obtaining data
___ 39. Ability to use computers for data collection and analysis
___ 40. Ability to recognize and explore a broad range of ideas and practices
___ 41. Ability to store data in an easily retrievable manner
___ 42. Ability to take complex ideas and processes and present them as models so that the models capture the complex processes
___ 43. Ability to review collections of written comments and pull out the common themes
___ 44. Ability to use basic statistical processes to make sense of data
___ 45. Ability to integrate diverse sources of data
___ 46. Ability to take complex data and reduce them to common themes and make sense of them
___ 47. Ability to do cost-benefit analysis

Data Presentation
___ 48. Ability to project trends and potential futures
___ 49. Ability to put together written reports regarding data and outcomes
___ 50. Ability to present data analysis using verbal communications skills
___ 51. Ability to manage questions placed to you
___ 52. Ability to select the appropriate AV materials for presentations
___ 53. Ability to work with groups and teams in presenting and discussing the data

Action Planning and Evaluation
___ 54. Ability to develop an action plan consisting of who, what, when, where, why, how much, and the desired outcomes
___ 55. Ability to monitor and track the progress of an action plan
___ 56. Ability to respond to changes and make midcourse corrections
___ 57. Ability to control anxiety while in the midst of a consultation
___ 58. Ability to design forms and inventories to aid in an evaluation
___ 59. Ability to feel comfortable with the client's review of your work
___ 60. Ability to terminate and have closure with a project

Action Planning
1. What key skills have you identified that you consider to be your strengths? List at least four.

2. What key skills have you identified as your weaknesses?

3. For each skill identified in question 2, identify what the next step would be for you to turn it into a strong skill.

4. How will you know when you have that skill developed? What will be different about the way you do your work, and how will that be useful for you?

10

Ethical Issues and Common Pitfalls

This chapter is about ethical issues and other pitfalls with which the internal consultant needs to be concerned. Why is a discussion of ethics important in a book on internal consulting? Very simply, internal consulting depends on trust. If the client loses trust in the consultant's integrity, the consultant is no longer effective. Assume for a moment that you are the internal consultant in the following setting.

> You are an internal consultant working with an external consultant. You have taken the external consultant to lunch and plan to expense that lunch to the organization.
> However, a day later, you and your boss go out for a social evening. It is purely social, and you are with several others for a fun night on the town. When it comes time to pay the tab, your boss turns to you and says, "Just put it on the expense tab for the lunch with the external consultant. Everyone does it—that is part of our culture here."

What is your response? What do you do? After all, he is your boss and is saying to go ahead, yet it is purely a social event. What would your decision be and why?

The above discussion is simply one part of the ethics discussion. What are the ethical pitfalls in internal consulting? How will you recognize an ethical issue when you meet one?

Ethical Issues and Common Pitfalls

This chapter will discuss ethical pitfalls. We will begin with a discussion of what ethics means in the context of the internal consultant and then discuss ethical issues at each stage of the process.

We have several important beliefs regarding the ethics of internal consulting. First, good ethics makes good business sense. Ethics is not something with which the internal consultant is concerned because he is a nice person. Ethics makes or breaks the internal consultant. Consider for a moment what would happen if the word got around the departments that you had betrayed a trust. Without a moment's hesitation, your work would come to a halt not just for this project but also for future ones.

Second, there are some areas where the ethical decision is clear, and there are others where the ethical decision requires a judgment call. It becomes a choice between values. That is why it is important for the internal consultant to be aware of her or his own value system, which forms the foundation of her or his system of ethics. In the midst of the decision of what to do, you can at least have the internal clarity of what is important for you. The internal consultant is a maker of value judgments when it comes to ethics.

Third, all decisions have some ethical component, although some are more ethically driven than others. Even, and perhaps most important, the decisions that drive the financial side of the organization are based on the ethics of the organization.

Fourth, ethical questions are the foundation for internal consulting. Remember, this is a helper-helpee relationship. That means that the helpee has some degree of dependency on the helper early in the relationship. The helper needs to be particularly sensitive to manipulations and inappropriate influencing that might occur in the relationship. The consultant has a degree of power and control over the client. That power and control need to be requested by the consultant.

The purpose of this chapter, then, is to approach ethics from the standpoint of decision making. Many of the tools discussed thus far might well be used in the making of decisions.

Our goal is to point to some of the ethical pitfalls and put up warnings.

Approaches: Means and Ends

Ethics is simply the study of what constitutes good and bad human conduct. It is looking at standards of behavior and conduct that have been judged "good" or "bad" by society. While at first this appears simple enough, further exploration demonstrates a complexity. Who determines what is good or bad conduct? What about the gray areas where there is no clear good or bad? What about intentions—if we have unintentional bad consequences, what does that mean? What if we have good results, but the way we got them was highly questionable?

As these questions indicate, we can begin to look at the question of ethics for the internal consultant in several ways. We can look at the consequences of behavior, following the rules, the means to the end, and the intentions.

The first approach considers the consequences of acts. Here we are concerned with the results and not with the intention of the internal consultant. Was the result the desired ethical one? This is a results-oriented approach. For example, the consultant may have been unsure about doing a particular something, but the outcome was excellent for those involved and the organization. What are considered are the consequences of the actions. Stated another way, the end justifies the means. Assume the following example.

> You are a consultant working with a department, and you find that the department has strong racial prejudices that impact some department members. The racial prejudices are open and overt. They include jokes, putdowns, and so on. While this observation is not related to the contract that you have with the department, you are concerned about it.
>
> You decide to violate the "trust" you have with the client and talk to human resources about the problem. The result is that the human resources department discusses

Ethical Issues and Common Pitfalls

your findings with the department manager's administrator, who then begins a study of the department. The department manager is reprimanded, and several employees are dismissed.

You choose to break the trust of the department manager to address an organizational issue. Does the end justify the means?

In this example the internal consultant found something unrelated to his project and reported on it. The end result was good for the organization. Again the key for us is the contract. During the initial contract there should be a discussion regarding what happens to the information collected during the course of the project. We include a clause stating that any information with negative organizational implications will be reported to administration. Ideally, the client would do the reporting. If not, we would report it, but this has to be part of the contract. In the earlier example of the inappropriate payment of the dinner tab, the key is not whether the internal consultant followed rules to determine whether or not to pick up the tab. The key is what happened as a result.

The second approach to ethics has to do with rules. Globally, these are rules that deal with the Golden Rule ("Do unto others as you would have them do unto you"). They are the accepted norms of behavior. This is a legalistic approach. The internal consultant has a specific set of rules to follow, and those determine ethical behavior or lack thereof. Consider the following example.

The client for whom you have been working demands that you provide him with names of employees who have indicated that they have made some personal phone calls from work. This came out in a study being done with regard to telephone usage, and the information was to be kept confidential. The manager of the area was surprised at the number of personal calls and wants to "discuss" this with the individuals involved.

You refuse because you believe strongly that since

you gathered the data with confidentiality of responses as a given, it would break a major norm of consulting work. Also, since the issue does not radically impact the organization, it is not one in which the organizational good overrides all else.

The accepted rules of behavior say that when information is gathered confidentially, unless something illegal or harmful to the organization is revealed, that confidentiality needs to be respected.

A third approach to ethics involves the means by which you arrive at a consequence. This is the traditional determination of whether means justify ends. This is a process orientation. Is the process one generally agreed on as a legitimate process? The key here is whether the means justify the ends. An end result that was achieved by questionable means becomes suspect. Consider the following example.

The internal consultant has just completed a project with a major client. There is a good deal of conflict regarding the final report. The client thinks that the internal consultant blew it, and the report is inaccurate. The internal consultant is accused of bias and not reporting the complete findings.

The internal consultant goes back to the process and walks through what was done step by step. Draft material from each is included. The result is reaffirmed.

A fourth approach to the ethics question is concerned with intention. What were your intentions? Did you intend to do harm? Did you intend to ignore the other person?

Part of the reason that we feel strongly with regard to the contracting and consulting process that we have outlined is that it contains integrity. In internal consulting work, there are many gray areas where the best we can do is say that we followed the process. The process itself becomes an important part of our professional integrity.

Our approach involves all three aspects—the intention,

Ethical Issues and Common Pitfalls

the means, and the ends. If any of these is out of balance, the question of ethics is raised. For example, if the intent is to defraud the organization by false billing, that is automatically an ethical issue (as well as a legal one). If the internal consultant uses questionable means to arrive at a desired end, that has ethical implications. If the internal consultant's intentions and means were good but the end result is questionable, that raises ethical questions.

Why Be Concerned with Ethics?

Why should we have a section in a book on internal consulting focused on the topic of ethics? Why is that important? We have indicated some reasons in this chapter, but we want to expand on them.

If we define ethics as good or bad human conduct, our discussion of ethics becomes very important. The work of the internal consultant is in the context of the helping relationship. If the internal consultant is perceived as being unethical, he or she will be ineffective in his or her work. Remember that the foundation for internal consulting is the helping relationship. If the internal consultant is perceived as unethical and, consequently, untrustworthy, the work will be ineffective. This is an approach that emphasizes the ends.

As a bottom line, the consulting process is built around valid information that is accurate. Questionable ethical conduct on the part of the consultant will erode valid and accurate information.

This means that good ethics is not a convenience for the internal consultant but is rather a given. Without ethics the internal consultant might as well close shop.

Why have a section on ethics? Because ethics makes good business sense!

Organizational Ethics. In the chapter on organizational culture, we discussed assumptions as being the foundation for the organizational culture. Within those basic assumptions are also assumptions that define ethical behavior. Remember our earlier assertion that there is an ethical component in all of our decisions. Whether or not we know or acknowledge it, there is a set of assumptions involving ethics that drive the decision making.

The start point for any discussion of ethics within an organization is this: Does the organization have a published policy or statement regarding ethical actions? What is the organization's statement regarding its employees' behavior? Do the following exercise.

Take a moment and think about your own organization. Is there a published statement or code of ethics? If you do not know, your human resources people may be able to help you. Or ask your chief administrator. Once you have gotten it, take time to read it over and see what it says. How does it sound to you? Hopefully, it sounds a bit pie in the sky.

Now think about the last time that the policy was quoted or used. What stories are there in the organization about individuals who took ethical stances? What happened to them? What are some settings in which you would like to see the policy used more?

If there is no published document, talk to some people about why. Do the same exercise as above but reflect on what the unpublished statement must say. Based on behavior you see around you, what is your hunch about how the document would read?

The second step at the organizational level is to look at the behavior of supervisors. A key influence on the ethical behavior of an employee is the response and backing of the supervisor. Think about the example that opened this chapter. That was a clear case where the supervisor was advocating breaking of a rule. Do the following exercise.

Think about yourself as supervisory. If you were to make a statement to your employees about ethics, what would you say to them? When you think of the statement you just made, what would be an example of an ethical issue that you recently handled that is consistent or inconsistent with that statement?

Now take a moment and think about your boss. What

Ethical Issues and Common Pitfalls

would your boss say to you about ethics? What does your boss's behavior say to you about ethics?

In the literature of social responsibility of organizations, there is an *iron law of responsibility* (Davis, Frederick, and Blomstrom, 1980, p. 50) that states that in the long run, those that do not use power in a way that society considers responsible will tend to lose it. We believe that is also true in the organization. Those who abuse power will tend to lose it. Managers who speak of but do not practice ethics may have short-run gains but long-run loses. Supervisors and managers need to recognize the importance of their modeling ethical behavior and what that communicates to the employees. The previous exercise is designed to help you look at your ethical behavior and your perception of your boss's.

Blanchard and Peale (1988) suggest five principles of ethical power in organizations that sum most of what we have been discussing regarding the organizational ethic.

First, organizations with high ethical standards need to communicate those through their mission statement and in their statement of purpose. The question, then, is: What is communicated from top management on down regarding ethics and expectations for ethical behavior? Think for a moment about your organization. What is communicated down from the top management regarding ethics?

Second, since organizational pride is a result of how people feel about themselves and the organization, organizational pride will be high when the employees feel that the organization's decisions are ethical and right. A quick way to undermine pride in an organization is to make decisions in a manner that employees consider questionable. How does pride in your organization influence you in making an ethical decision?

Think about your organization. What is a decision that employees had to implement that they thought was questionable? What was the impact? What is a decision the employees had to implement of which they were proud? What was the impact?

Third, an organization must be patient. This means that the organization is unwilling to make short-term gains inconsistent with their value core at the cost of long-term interests. Within health care organizations this is a significant perspective. Frequently, the pressures are on to make short-term decisions that bring into question the long-term organizational values. The question is: How does the patience or impatience of your organization impact your ability to make an ethical decision? Take a few moments and think about how patient or impatient your organization is. What is the impact on your ethical decision making?

Fourth, an organization must have persistence. Persistence means doing what you say you are going to do. The leadership of the organization sticks to what it says it is going to do. The question is: How does your organization's persistence facilitate you when you face an ethical dilemma?

What is an example of where your organization changed its mind and did not carry through on something that it said it would do? What was the impact? What is an example of where your organization carried through on what it said it was going to do? What was the impact here?

Fifth, an organization must have perspective. Managers and administration need to take time to reflect on where they are and where they are going. There is a sense of managed growth and change. Employees are expected to take a step back and reflect on decisions. The question is: How does your organization facilitate or hinder taking time to reflect on ethical dilemmas?

Think about your organization. What are the organization's expectations of you? Are you expected to take time and think about the ethical dilemmas? If so, what was one of the last ethical dilemmas, and how did you think it through?

The first step is the organizational ethic. The organizational ethic provides the container in which individual ethical decisions are made. If the organization has clear ethical statements and intents, the message will carry down the organization. If the organization is muddy and unclear regarding ethics,

Ethical Issues and Common Pitfalls

Exhibit 13. Organizational Ethical Audit.

1. Obtain a copy of the ethical conduct statement for your organization. Read it over. What does it say to you regarding ethical conduct?
2. Think about the major organizational decisions in the past year. What are the messages that these decisions send to the organization with regard to top management's views of ethics?
3. What are some of the stories regarding ethics in your organization? Who was fired or reprimanded for a breach of ethics? Who was not fired or reprimanded for a breach of ethics?
4. When you think about your organization, are you proud of its ethics? When you are in public, are you proud to be associated with the organization?
5. Does top management take ethics seriously? Or is ethics considered to be anti–bottom line? What are your data here?

---

this will carry down the organization. Exhibit 13 provides some additional questions for doing an organizational ethics audit.

Personal Ethics. Any discussion of ethics needs to take into account the individual's background and ethical system. Remember our discussion in Chapter Two regarding percept language? The foundation for our individual ethics is filter 2—the learnings and experiences of our past. Each of us carries in us values about what is good and bad behavior. Each of us carries an ethical system.

This means that in any organizational setting, the various organizational members have their own beliefs about ethics. The more diverse the organization, the more diverse the responses to the individual ethics.

It is important for internal consultants to be aware of their own ethical standards and the standards of the profession. The following questions attempt to create some of that awareness.

1. Recall some event in your recent past when you said to yourself, "That person acted unethically." What was the behavior to which you objected?

2. When you think about the behavior to which you objected, what value(s) do you hold that was (were) offended?
3. If you were to write a statement of belief about ethics, what would it be? Take a few minutes and do it.
4. Review your statement in question 3. When was the last time you acted on that statement? What was the setting?

The organization is a collection of individuals with a variety of ethical beliefs and values. However, the organization attracts certain individuals because the organizational ethics and personal ethics match. A function of the recruitment and selection process is to formally and informally let the candidates know the ethical expectations. Those who do not fit with the organization will not join it or will become uncomfortable enough to eventually leave.

Professional Ethics. The organization has an ethics, and the individual has an ethics. However, it is an important point to make clear that there is also a professional ethics. Each of us in health care has professional organizations with which we are associated, be it nursing, pharmacy, education, business office, marketing, or whatever. Many of those organizations have their own code of conduct or code of ethics. Think about the professional organizations of which you are part. Do they have a published code of conduct?

Lippitt and Lippitt (1986, pp. 85–87) suggest that the foundation of any professional role is:

1. acquiring the knowledge and learnings necessary for that role
2. learning to apply professional knowledge and learnings to real-life settings
3. always putting client needs first
4. maintaining high standards
5. behaving at all times with professional bearing

Based on this foundation, a profession is built. Key to that building is a code of ethics. Lippitt and Lippitt continue on to

Ethical Issues and Common Pitfalls

suggest a code of ethics that might apply to consulting work. We have included here only those items that apply to internal consulting.

Code of Ethics for the Professional Consultant.

1. *Responsibility*. The consultant places high value on objectivity and integrity and maintains the highest standards of service and plans work in a way that minimizes the possibility of misleading findings.

2. *Competence*. The consultant maintains high standards of professional competence as a responsibility to the public and to the profession, recognizes the boundaries of his or her competence and does not offer services that fail to meet professional standards, assists clients in obtaining professional help for aspects of the projects that fall outside the boundaries of his or her own competence, and refrains from undertaking any activity in which his or her personal problems are likely to result in inferior professional service or harm to the client.

3. *Moral and legal standards*. The consultant shows sensible regard for the social codes and moral expectations of the community in which he or she works.

4. *Misrepresentation*. The consultant avoids misrepresentations of her or his professional qualifications, affiliations, and purposes and those of the organization with which she or he is associated.

5. *Confidentiality*. The consultant reveals information received in confidence to only the appropriate authorities, maintains confidentiality of professional conjunctions about individuals, informs the client of the limits of confidentiality, and maintains confidentiality in preservation and disposition of records.

6. *Client welfare*. The consultant defines the nature of his or her loyalties and responsibilities in possible conflicts of interest, such as between the client and the consultant's employer, and keeps all concerned parties informed of these commitments; attempts to terminate a consulting relationship when it is reasonably clear that the client is not benefiting from it; and continues being responsible for the welfare of the client, in cases

involving referral, until the responsibility is assumed by the professional to whom the client is referred or until the relationship with the client has been terminated by mutual agreement.

7. *Intraprofessional and interprofessional relations.* The consultant acts with integrity toward colleagues in consultation and in other professions.

8. *Responsibility toward organization.* The consultant respects the rights and reputation of the organization with which she or he is associated.

9. *Promotional activities.* The consultant, when associated with the development or promotion of products offered for commercial sale, ensures that the products are presented in a factual way.

The Organization plus the Personal Ethic

We have carried on a general discussion regarding ethics. What practical steps can the internal consultant consider during the consultation process to identify an ethical question? Davis, Frederick, and Blomstrom (1980, p. 213) suggest that the following questions be asked:

1. *Is there unfair gain to the person doing it?* Does someone benefit unduly from the transaction? The trick is the definition of "unfair gain." In a particular setting, it often is relatively easy to determine that a person gains some great advantage. If so, the question of ethics needs to be considered.

2. *Is there unfair harm to others?* Again, the question of unfair harm comes to mind. While in some settings it is useful to define unfair harm, in other settings it is a matter of sensing. Again, if unfair harm occurs, an ethical question may be involved.

3. *How substantial is the harm or gain?* Relating to the two previous questions is how severe or significant the gain or harm is. The more severe or significant, the more questionable it becomes.

4. *Was the action based on a personal decision, or was the action representative of an established practice?* This is a critical question. Whenever a decision is based on pure personal choice rather

Ethical Issues and Common Pitfalls

Exhibit 14. Ethical Guides for Personal Action.

---

1. Identify a recent ethical dilemma that you have had:

2. Now identify three courses of action you could have taken to address this ethical issue.
   A.

   B.

   C.

3. For each of the above courses of action, ask the following questions:
   a. Is the action legal?
   b. Is there unfair gain to the person doing it? How substantial is the gain?
   c. Is there unfair harm to others? How substantial is the harm?
   d. Is the action based on personal decision or established practices?
   e. Is there a due process?
   f. How would the decision make you feel about yourself? If it were made public, would you feel proud of it?
4. Based on your thinking, the "best" choice would be:

---

than an established process, the potential for an ethical conflict exists. For example, in the work of the internal consultant, the internal consulting process represents a guide for the conduct of business. If the consultant is clear about following the process, there is less chance for unethical behavior.

5. *Is there adequate due process?* Is there an opportunity for the parties involved to appeal a particular decision or to get additional information into the system?

These questions can be used as a guide for looking at a particular decision and deciding whether an ethical issue exists. Exhibit 14 is a questionnaire designed to assist you in working on ethical decisions.

A second useful approach to identifying ethical issues that is very simple to use was developed by Blanchard and Peale

(1988). They pose three questions for the manager (or in our case, the internal consultant).

First, is the decision that you are looking at legal in both civil law and company policy? If we refer back to the opening case, the response would be that the action would not pass this particular criterion. Therefore, it would be unethical and probably illegal to do.

Second, is the decision balanced and fair to all concerned in the long run? Does it promote opportunities for the parties involved to succeed?

Third, how does this decision make you feel about yourself? If it were published on the front page of a newspaper, would you be proud of it? If it were announced to your family, would you be pleased?

Based on the responses to these three questions, we arrive at whether or not a particular decision is ethical, or we can at least begin to reach this decision. This approach provides the internal consultant with a quick and efficient way to determine if a decision is ethical or not.

One last comment here. We want to present you with a system that can be used as an ethical guide, but we do not want to minimize a significant issue. Many times questions open more questions than they answer. That is to be expected, because most ethical issues are not easily resolved. They are questions that pit values against values. These questions can be used as a framework for decisions.

Ethical Pitfalls

Each stage of the consulting process that was overviewed in Chapter Three has associated ethical pitfalls for which to watch. These are places where ethical questions might arise. The major ones that we have identified include:

Contracting and Precontracting. There are two major categories of ethical dilemmas—those related to the ability to do the work and those related to relationship.

A major ethical dilemma is whether to say yes to a project

Ethical Issues and Common Pitfalls

that either you are not competent to do or with which you have a value conflict. The tendency can be to take on a project with which you are unfamiliar without letting the client know your status. This last sentence is key.

We do not see an ethical problem if you tell the client that you have not done this type of project before but are willing to do it now. The client has full information and can decide for himself or herself. The problem is when the client is left with the assumption that the project is something of a type with which you are familiar.

The other type of pitfall involves taking on a project with which you have a value conflict without informing the client of that conflict. You may disagree with how the client will use the information that you are gathering. Whatever the case, it is important to let the client know of your value conflict and, if the conflict is significant enough, to not take the consult.

Here are a number of other client problems. You might give the client false information about who you are or what you have done. This relates to the first but is broader in nature. It may include giving unrealistic expectations to the client.

1. *Not giving the client full information.* For example, if you have severe doubts about the project and you do not state these, you are withholding information that is important for the client.

2. *Taking on projects that are not in line with the good of the organization.* Such a project may result in the client's winning but the organization's losing.

3. *Making impossible agreements.* This involves setting or agreeing to impossible objectives. This is known as a setup for failure. There is no way that there can be a "win."

4. *Not arriving at an agreement on confidentiality and what that means in this context.* Confidentiality means many things to many different people. It is important to specify what it means in this context. We have found it important to talk to the client regarding confidentiality. If while working with a client we find information vital to the organization, we will share that information with the appropriate managers. Remember, our primary client is the organization.

Data Collection and Analysis. Some of the ethical dilemmas to be alert to in data collection and analysis include:

1. *Collecting information not needed or required.* Avoid asking unneeded questions. It is a waste of time and energy for all parties.

2. *Using methods inappropriate for the data being collected.* This implies incompetence. It means not using the tools of collection or analysis appropriately.

3. *Doing inappropriate editing of the comments or the data to please or avoid displeasure of a client.*

4. *Not sharing with the client the limitations of the collection or data analysis.* This can result in a false data valuation. There needs to be a clear statement of the shortcomings of the collection process and the analysis process.

Data Presentation. Some pitfalls during data presentation include:

1. *Misrepresenting the data.* This results in the client's having poor information to make a decision. The client leaves with something worse than no information—misinformation.

2. *Withholding from the client.* The internal consultant may decide to withhold certain information. Again, this can mean that the client leaves without good information for decision making.

3. *Sharing of confidential information.* Information may be inappropriately shared prior to, during, or after the presentation with inappropriate parties.

4. *Not sharing organizational information that has significant impact on the organization with the proper authorities.* Remember that your ultimate client is the organization. This means that key impacts on the organization need to be shared with decision makers.

Action Plan. Some pitfalls with the action plan are:

1. *Setting impossible or unattainable targets.* This is a carryover from contracting. The targets set may simply not be reasonable.

Ethical Issues and Common Pitfalls

2. *Not being clear about expectations.* Again, this repeats earlier comments.

3. *Withholding information.* Clearly this is key. If information is withheld, the plan can totally miss its mark.

Evaluation. Some pitfalls during evaluation include:

1. *Withholding information.* This might be an unwillingness to share negative data. It can be hard at the end of a long, time-consuming, and resource-consuming consult to say, "We did not get it done."

2. *Using the data in inappropriate ways.* Frequently, there will be interest on the part of others in what is happening with the consult. Coffee discussions or lunch breaks will be a time when someone might say, "By the way, what is happening with that project?"

These represent some pitfalls in the various steps of the internal consulting process. Note the two themes that are important throughout. The first and most important is keeping valid information flowing. This means keeping the client fully informed of key information that will impact him or her. Regardless of the phase of consulting, that valid information is crucial. It is the lifeblood of the consult. Second, be aware of your own competencies and limitations and plan accordingly.

Summary

For the internal consultant, ethics is not just something nice to do. It is the vital foundation. Without a clear sense of the ethical implications of the role of the internal consultant, the internal consultant can do significant damage to the organization, the event with which he or she is working, and himself or herself.

11

The Keys to Successful Internal Consulting

Learning Keys

Our purpose in writing this book is simple—to increase productivity and performance of individuals in health care organizations by providing them a set of skills known as internal consulting. Health care organizations have a unique environment that makes the use of internal consultants even more important. Health care organizations are labor-intensive organizations that require high levels of people interaction and teamwork to get to the desired result of high-quality patient care. The solution proposed throughout this book is the internal consulting role.

The organization that accepts our challenge will build on the current technical skills of its health care professionals. The goal will be to skill those health care professionals in the internal consulting process.

Some of the key points of the chapters of this book are:

Key 1. There are many ways to live out the role of internal consultant. The four key roles that we have proposed are director, counselor, facilitator, and delegator. Our thesis is that role selection depends on the situation in which the consultant is. Different conditions will require different behaviors of the consultant. At times she will need to be directive and at others facilitative.

The Keys to Successful Internal Consulting 247

Key 2. The consulting relationship is one of helper and helpee. The client is someone seeking help, and the consultant is someone offering help. This help can be in terms of assistance with problem solving, decision making, or presentation of future problems.

We believe it is vital for the internal consultant to recognize this helper-helpee relationship. At the core of the helping relationship is the need for the internal consultant to understand what it means for the client to be helped and for the internal consultant to be a helper.

Key 3. The consulting process is essentially a blueprint that directs the internal consultant. The process of internal consulting provides the internal consultant with benchmarks. By following the process he or she increases the probability of having a successful consultation. The steps of the process are:

1. *Precontracting.* This is the earliest contact between the consultant and the client. The consultant obtains information on the project and decides whether to continue or terminate the project.

2. *Contracting.* Perhaps the single most important step in the process is establishing and clarifying tasks and relationships. This process is what we refer to as contracting. Contracting defines what needs to be done to meet the client's expectations. It defines the roles and who will do what during the process. The relationship is defined.

3. *Data collection.* The consultation process depends on good data. Without good data the process is little more than guessing. Data collection efforts focus on what needs to be collected, by what methods, and from what sources. We have provided various data collection tools and hints on using those tools.

4. *Data analysis.* Data gathering is one thing. Data analysis is another. The end product of the data collection is only as good as the analysis process. We have provided hints on quantitative and qualitative data analysis. The issues from the data analysis should ideally be ones that the client has control in changing,

are important for the organization, and have organizational commitment.

5. *Data presentation.* The work of the previous steps can be lost if the presentation is not well done. The goal of the presentation is to present a clear, concise, objective snapshot of the data. This allows the client to make the decision about next steps.

6. *Action planning.* The problem has been defined. Now it is time for the next steps. Action planning provides the structure in which the desired results are achieved. Action planning identifies who will do what, when, and with how many resources. The keys to action planning are solid contracting and data collection analysis.

7. *Evaluation.* Finally comes the question: How did we do? Did we get done what needed to get done? Or are serious parts of the contract left undone?

Evaluation is a time of asking these and other questions. It is a time of determining the value of the project. Has the consultant met the terms of the contract in the most effective, efficient manner possible?

8. *Termination.* Once again, remember that we have defined the internal consultant–client relationship as that of helper and helpee. That means that when the project is done, there will be a termination involving the task and the relationship. Termination means finding the most effective way of saying good-bye to the client for this time. That means that there is less of a tendency to have "unfinished business" from the past cloud the new project in future work.

Key 4. Organizational culture provides the context for the work of the consultant. Culture puts limits on how the consulting process and the internal consultant behave. Awareness of the culture and its strengths and limitations will enhance the consultant's abilities to work efficiently in the culture. We provide a number of recommendations on how to access the organization's culture and its possible impact on your work.

Key 5. Good ethics is a necessity for the internal consultant. In fact, without good ethics the consultant is probably

The Keys to Successful Internal Consulting 249

going to be without work. The reputation of the consultant as having integrity and being trustworthy is the vital foundation to the consultant's work. The consulting process is built around valid, accurate information. Valid information is obtained from a client who trusts.

Key 6. Internal consulting has a specific set of skills that are important for the internal consultant. We have identified those skills throughout this book. The next section is designed to take the skills one step further.

Transitions: Where to Go for More

What now? Suppose you have decided that we are right and you want to skill yourself in internal consulting skills. What is your next step?

We have several suggestions. The first set are places you might look in your organization, and the second set are places you might look outside your organization.

First, within your organization, we suggest:

1. Look at others in the organization who might have internal consulting skills. There may be a person in human resources, education, or administration who has skills and would be willing to help you develop your skills.

2. Find out if there are consultants coming into your organization who might have skills that you need. Take them to lunch or coffee and ask them if they will work with you.

Outside of the organization, we suggest:

1. Look around to other industries. There may be another industry that has a person with internal consulting skills, and that person might be willing to assist you. We have found this to be an invaluable resource.

2. Visit colleges and universities and see who is doing consulting. Talk with these individuals about assisting you in developing your consulting skills. Again, this is a group that we have found very useful.

3. When you attend your professional meetings, look at the agenda for workshops that address internal consulting skills.

Many professional organizations have sessions at their professional meetings that relate to internal consulting skills.

4. Watch the mail for workshops that relate to consulting skills. If you do not get that type of mail, your education or human resources person probably does. Two major consulting organizations that provide both workshops and written materials are the National Training Labs (NTH) (1240 N. Pitt St. Centre, Ste. 100, Alexandria, Va. 22314) and University Associates (8517 Production Ave., San Diego, Calif. 92121). These two groups provide excellent resources for developing internal consultant skills.

Summary

As we walked through the internal consulting model, we introduced and reviewed skills for each component. Our goal was that you would end the journey with knowledge, wisdom, and skills about the role of the internal consultant. For some of you we were walking on new territory; for others it was a trip down memory lane. In whatever situation you found yourself, we hope that you found it useful and insightful.

As the health care industry continues its growth and change, we are confident that the role of the internal consultant will continue to grow and be empowered, as it is one way that we can respond to key issues that plague the health care industry today.

Ideally, from reading our book, you have begun building the foundation necessary for internal consulting in the health care industry. The challenge for each of us is to build on existing skills and obtain new skills to facilitate our transition into the world of successful consulting. Empowering oneself through such skilling is the first step in the desired direction. As one builds on successful consulting experiences and learns from the unsuccessful ones, it becomes a natural part of the everyday work life. As we begin to identify ourselves as internal consultants, we will begin to model the role to others in the organization. Hopefully, the organization will experience the increase in effectiveness, and the end result will be a more effective team working together toward the end result—quality patient care.

References

Adizes, I. *Corporate Life Cycles.* Englewood Cliffs, N. J.: Prentice-Hall, 1988.

Argyris, C. *Intervention Theory and Method: A Behavioral Science Point of View.* Reading, Mass.: Addison-Wesley, 1973.

Austin, E. *Guidelines for the Development of Continuing Education Offerings for Nurses.* New York: Appleton-Century-Crofts, 1981.

Ball, G. *Using Graphics with Groups.* Palo Alto, Calif.: Process Management Associates, 1978.

Barney, J. "Organizational Culture: Can It Be a Source of Sustained Competitive Advantage?" *Academy of Management Review,* July 1986, *11* (3), 656.

Blanchard, K., and Peale, N. V. *The Power of Ethical Management.* Escondido, Calif.: Blanchard Training and Development, 1988.

Block, P. *Flawless Consulting.* San Diego, Calif.: University Associates, 1981.

Brandt, R. *Flip Charts: How to Draw Them and How to Use Them.* Richmond, Va.: Brandt Management Group, 1986.

Bureau of Labor Statistics. *Monthly Review,* Sept. 1987.

Consultation Skills Inventory. In *1976 Annual Handbook for Group Facilitators.* San Diego, Calif.: University Associates, 1976.

Davis, K., Frederick, W., and Blomstrom, R. *Business and Society.* New York: McGraw-Hill, 1980.

Dunham, R. B., and Smith, F. J. *Surveys from Start to Finish.* Organizational Surveys: An Internal Assessment of Organizational Health, Info Line. Alexandria, Va.: American Society For Training and Development, 1979.

Fitz-Gibbon, C. T., and Morris, L. L. *How to Calculate Statistics.* Beverly Hills, Calif.: Sage, 1979.

Hackett, T. "The Real Role of Personnel Managers." *Personnel Journal.* Mar. 1988, pp. 70ff.

Hersey, P., and Blanchard, K. *Management of Organizational Behavior.* Englewood Cliffs, N. J.: Prentice-Hall, 1977.

Hersey, P., and Natemeyer, W. *Power Perception Profile.* San Diego, Calif.: Center for Leadership Studies, University Associates, 1979.

"Into the Twenty-First Century." Bethesda, Md.: World Future Society, 1988.

Jones, J. "The Sensing Interview." In *1973 Annual Handbook for Group Facilitators.* San Diego, Calif.: University Associates, 1973.

Jones, J. "Meeting Management: Coping with Dysfunctional Behaviors." In *1986 Annual: Developing Human Resources.* San Diego, Calif.: University Associates, 1986.

Jones, J., and Bearley, W. *Group Development Assessment Questionnaire.* Bryn Mawr, Pa.: Organizational Design and Development, 1986.

Jones, J., and Pfeiffer, W. *1973 Annual Handbook for Group Facilitators.* San Diego, Calif.: University Associates, 1973.

Kelly, D., and Conner, D. "The Emotional Change Cycle." In *1979 Annual Handbook for Group Facilitators.* San Diego, Calif.: University Associates, 1979.

Lawrence, P., and Lorsch, J. *Developing Organizations: Diagnosis and Action.* Reading, Mass.: Addison-Wesley, 1969.

Lewin, K. *A Dynamic Theory of Personality.* New York: McGraw-Hill, 1935.

Lippitt, G., and Lippitt, R. *The Consulting Process in Action.* San Diego, Calif.: University Associates, 1986.

Luft, J., and Ingham, H. "Johari Window: A Model for Soliciting and Giving Feedback." In *1973 Annual Handbook for Group Facilitators.* San Diego, Calif.: University Associates, 1973.

McGregor, D. "The Human Side of Enterprise." *Management Review,* Nov. 1957.

References

McLagan, P. *Models for Excellence: The Conclusions and Recommendations of the ASTD Training and Development Competency Study.* Washington, D. C.: American Society for Training and Development, 1983.

Maehr, M., and Braskamp, L. *The Motivational Factor: A Theory of Personal Investment.* Lexington, Mass.: Lexington Books, 1986.

Margulies, N., and Raia, A. P. *Conceptual Foundations of Organizational Development.* New York: McGraw-Hill, 1978.

Nadler, D. "Organizational Analysis, Design and Implementation: An Approach for Improving Effectiveness." In *1983 Annual for Facilitators, Trainers and Consultants.* San Diego, Calif.: University Associates, 1983.

Nolan, T. *Initial Client Contact.* 1982.

Peters, J., and Mabry, E. "The Personnel Officer as Internal Consultant." *Personnel Administrator*, Apr. 1981, pp. 29ff.

Polit, D., and Hungler, B. *Nursing Research: Principles and Methods.* Philadelphia: Lippincott, 1978.

Schein, E. H. *Organizational Culture and Leadership: A Dynamic View.* San Francisco: Jossey-Bass, 1985.

Scherer, J. In J. J. Sherwood and J. J. Scherer, "A Model for Couples: How Two Can Grow Together," *Journal for Small Group Behavior*, Feb. 1975. (Originally J. Gidewell and J. Sherwood, "Planned Renegotiation," in *Group Facilitators Handbook.* San Diego, Calif.: University Associates, 1973.)

Schutz, W. *The Truth Option.* Berkeley, Calif.: Ten Speed Press, 1984.

Scriven, M. "Evaluation Model." In Worthen, B., and Sanders, J. R. (eds.), *Education Evaluation: Theory and Practice.* Belmont, Calif.: Wadsworth, 1973.

SnowAntle, S., Stone, D., Vincelette, J., and Michaels, C. "Turnover Prediction—How to Use Employee Perception Data to Foresee Trends of the Workforce." *Personnel Administrator*, June 1989, pp. 146–148.

State of Florida Health Care Cost Containment Board, Department of Health and Rehabilitative Services. Annual Report. Tallahassee, Fla., 1988.

Stufflebeam, D. L. "Evaluation as Enlightenment for Decision Making." In Worthen, B., and Sanders, J. R. (eds.), *Education*

Evaluation: Theory and Practice. Belmont, Calif.: Wadsworth, 1973a.

Stufflebeam, D. L. "Evaluation Model." In Worthen, B., and Sanders, J. R. (eds.), *Education Evaluation: Theory and Practice.* Belmont, Calif.: Wadsworth, 1973b.

Ulschak, F. L. "Letting the Problem Do the Talking: A Systems Framework." *Transactional Analysis Journal,* Apr. 1978, *8* (2), 148-173.

Ulschak, F. L. "Creating the Future of Health and Education." Chicago: American Hospital Publishing, 1988.

Ulschak, F. L. "Corporate Culture: The Impact on Productivity and Performance." In McDougall, M., Covert, R., and Melton, V. B. (eds.), *Productivity and Performance Management in Healthcare Institutions.* Chicago: American Hospital Publishing, 1989.

Ulschak, F. L., Nathanson, L., and Gillan, P. *Small Group Problem Solving: An Aid to Organizational Effectiveness.* Reading, Mass.: Addison-Wesley, 1981.

Ulschak, F. L., and SnowAntle, S. Unpublished Delphi study of future health care trends. *Journal of the American Society of Healthcare Education and Training,* American Hospital Association, forthcoming.

Weir, J., and Weir, J. *Percept Language.* San Luis Obispo, Calif.: Weir Labs, 1985.

Windsor, R., and others. *Evaluation of Health Promotion and Education Programs.* Mountain View, Calif.: Mayfield, 1984.

Index

A

Accountability, 154
Action plan, 63; checklist, 162; and computer assistance, 150; costs, 147, 149; and ethics, 244–245; evaluation of, 153; objective, 145, 148–149; resources, 146–147, 149; responsibility, 146, 149; task dates, 146, 149; tasks to complete, 145, 149
Adizes, I., 187
Administrators, 12–13
Advance materials, 131
Advocate, 39
Agenda, 131, 138–140
Aging populations, 15
Ancillary departments, 10–11
Argyris, C., 75
Assumptions, 173–174, 175–177
Audiovisual equipment, 133–136
Austin, E., 136

B

Ball, G., 135
Barney, J., 180
Bearley, W., 46
Beepers, 136, 207
Bias, 133
Blanchard, K., 42, 235, 241–242
Blind spots, 33, 34, 35, 200

Block, P., 121, 126
Blomstrom, R., 235, 240
Brainstorming, 214
Brandt, R., 135
Braskamp, L., 86

C

Change, 16–17; emotional, cycle, 23–25; model, 21–23; and organizational culture, 178, 179–180, 187–191; resistance to, 22–23
Client: choices, 75; commitment, 75; defensiveness, 133; dependency, 49; identification, 13–14, 74–75; involvement, 132, 138, 140; welfare, 239–240
Closed-ended questions, 104–105
Closure. *See* Termination
Commitment, 86, 88; client, 75; and conflict management, 206; and influence, 201; and organizations, 172; and presentation, 130
Competence, 239
Computer software, 123, 150
Confidentiality, 93–94, 102, 158, 232, 239, 243
Conflict management, 202–210; cycle, 203–205
Conner, D., 23
Consultant, 7–8; external, 19–21, 56–57, 160, 185–186; process,

41-42. *See also* Internal consulting
Consultation Skills Inventory, 38, 225
Contracting, 61-62; checklist, 98; and confidentiality, 93-94; and contracts, 92-93; and CPR+F model, 85-91; and ethics, 242-243; and evaluation, 152-153, 154; and information, 91-92; pitfalls, 94-95; and presentation, 131-132; as process, 76; and relationship, 82-85; and task, 80-82; as tool, 76-77
Control behavior, 83, 84
Cost: containment, 15; evaluation, 160; project, 147, 149
Counselor role, 44, 45, 48
CPR+F model, 85-91; and influence, 201-202; and organizations, 170-173; and presentation, 130
Culture, organizational, 169-170; and change, 178, 179-180, 187-191; and CPR+F model, 170-173; defined, 173-178; identifying, 184-187; and internal consultant, 181-187; life cycle of, 187-191; and subcultures, 180, 182-183; transparency of, 179

D

Data analysis, 62, 99-101, 121; checklist, 128; and ethics, 244; qualitative, 121-123; quantitative, 122, 123-126
Data collection, 62, 99-101; checklist, 128; and ethics, 244; by interviews, 107-111; by observation, 111-114; by questionnaires, 102-107; by reports and records, 114-116; by sensing group, 116-121
Data presentation. *See* Presentation
Davis, K., 235, 240
Delegator role, 44-45, 49
Dependency, of client, 49
Directiveness, 39, 42

Director role, 44, 45, 48
Dunham, R. B., 104

E

Education and training, 9-10
Educator, 40-41
Emotional change cycle, 23-25
Environment, 172
Ethics, 93, 183, 228-230; and consequences, 230-231; and intentions, 232; organizational, 233-237; personal, 237-238, 240-242; pitfalls, 242-245; professional, 238-240; and rules, 231-232
Evaluation, 63, 151-152; checklist, 162; and contract, 152-153, 154; design, 157-160; and ethics, 245; formative, 156-157; purposes of, 152-154; summative, 156-157; and termination, 154, 162-164
External consultants, 19-21, 56-57, 160, 185-186

F

Facilitator role, 44, 45, 48-49
Fact finder, 41
Feedback, 87, 89; and conflict management, 206; and influence, 201; and organizations, 172; and presentation, 130. *See also* Presentation
First impressions, 59, 60
Fitz-Gibbon, C. T., 123, 126
Flip charts, 134-135
Follow-up: action plan, 147; presentation, 141-142
Force field analysis, 216-218
Formative evaluation, 156-157
Frederick, W., 235, 240

G

Generalization, 153
Gillan, P., 213
Gantt chart, 146
Group, sensing, 116-121

Index

H

Hackett, T., 10
Hawthorne effect, 112
Health care organizations: characteristics of, 4; departments in, 8-13; effectiveness of, 4-5, 14; trends affecting, 14-17. *See also* Culture, organizational
Health care professionals, shortages of, 16
Helper-helpee role, 28-29, 33
Hersey, P., 42, 197
Human resources (HR), 10

I

Inclusion behavior, 83, 84
Influence, 196-202
Information, 75, 91-92; and evaluation, 157-159, 160-161; and organizational culture, 183-184; and power, 198; resources, 9; specialist, 39-40; transfer, 5-6. *See also* Data analysis; Data collection; Presentation
Ingham, H., 33
Integrity, 232
Interdependency, 5
Internal consulting: checklist, 226-227; criteria, 12; defined, 7-8; departments involved in, 8-13; ethical code, 239-240; ethical pitfalls, 242-245; and external consulting, 21, 56-57; minuses of, 18-19; and organizational culture, 181-187; primary, roles, 42-49; process, 57-64; skills, 4, 6; strengths of, 17-18
Interviews, 107-111; and culture identification, 187; group, 116-121
"Into the Twenty-First Century," 14-15
Investment, 86

J

Johari window, 33-35, 196
Joint problem solver, 41
Jones, J., 46, 116, 223

K

Kelly, D., 23

L

Lawrence, P., 117
Lewin, K., 21, 216
Linking role, 41
Lippitt, G., 39, 45-46, 238
Lippitt, R., 39, 45-46, 238
Listening, 194-196; and conflict management, 208
Lorsch, J., 117
Luft, J., 33

M

Mabry, E., 10
McGregor, D., 176
McLagan, P., 38, 225
Maehr, M., 86
Managers, 12-13
Margulies, N., 36
Marketing, 11
MaxThink, 123
Mean, 124-126
Median, 125-126
Metaphors, 224
Michaels, C., 16
Microsoft Project, 150
Morris, L. L., 123, 126

N

Nadler, D., 151
Natemeyer, W., 197
Nathanson, L., 213
National Training Labs (NTL), 250
Needs, 29, 46
Networking, 41
Nolan, T., 58
Nominal group process, 218-222
Nondirective, 39
Nonverbal communication, 109, 119, 194-195
Norms, 173
Nursing, 11-12

O

Objective, 145, 148–149
Objectivity, 132–133
Observation, 111–114
Open-ended questions, 104
Openness behavior, 83, 84
Organizations. *See* Culture, organizational; Ethics: organizational; Health care organizations
Overhead tranparencies, 134

P

Pastoral care, 11
Peale, N. V., 235, 241–242
Percept language model, 31–33
Perceptions, 31–35, 82
Peters, J., 10
Pinch model, 77–80
Power bases, 197–201
Precontracting, 58–61; checklist, 98; and ethics, 242–243
Premeeting planning form, 137
Presentation, 62–63; and audiovisual equipment, 133–136; checklist, 143; and CPR + F model, 130; and ethics, 244; follow-up, 141–142; group, meeting, 138–141; one-on-one, meeting, 138; and premeeting planning form, 137; preparation, 130–138; process, 129–130; report, 138, 140
Problem: identification, 8, 80–82, 99–100; and organizational culture, 181–182; types, 29–30, 210–213. *See also* Problem solving
Problem solving: process, 213–222; suggestions, 222–224; and types of problems, 210–213
Process consultant, 41–42
Process orientation, 36–37, 38
Productivity, 4–5
Psychosocial medicine, 11
Public relations (PR), 11
Purpose, 85–86, 88–89; and conflict management, 206; and influence, 201; and organizations, 170, 172; and presentation, 130

Q

Questionnaires, 102–107; and culture identification, 187

R

Raia, A. P., 36
Random selection, 103
Rating scales, 105–106
Records, 114–116. *See also* Information
Refreezing, 23
Regulation, 16
Reimbursement, 14, 16
Relationship, 42–43; defining, 82–85; in interviews, 108; and pinch model, 77–80; termination, 162–164
Reliability testing, 103
Reports: and data collection, 114–116; presentation, 132, 138, 140; structure of, 133. *See also* Information
Resistance, 22–23, 119
Resources, project, 146–147, 149
Responsibility: ethical, 235, 239; project, 146, 149
Roles: choosing among, 45–49; and conflict management, 206; and CPR + F model, 86, 89, 130, 172; helper-helpee, 28–29, 33; and influence, 201; multiple, 35–42; and organizational culture, 183–184; and organizations, 172; and presentation, 130; primary, 42–45; shifting, 49, 51

S

Schein, E. H., 20–21, 175
Scherer, J., 77
Schutz, W., 83
Scouting, 60
Scriven, M., 156
Self-care, 16
Self-understanding, 31, 33
Sensing group, 116–121
Situational leadership, 42

Index

Skunk works, 183
Slides, 134
Smith, F. J., 104
SnowAntle, S., 16, 154
Stamp collecting, 79
Standard deviation, 126
Statistics, 123-124; descriptive, 124-126; and evaluation, 158-159; inferential, 126; uses and abuses of, 126-127
Stone, D., 16
Stufflebeam, D. L., 156, 157
Subcultures, 180, 182-183
Summative evaluation, 156-157

T

Task: and action plan, 145-146, 149; defining, 80-82; orientation, 36, 37-38
Teamwork, 47-48
Technical expert, 38-39
Technical skills, 4, 6
Technological change, 15
Termination, 63-64, 154, 162-164

Theme list, 122
Theory X/Theory Y, 176
Time factor, 46-47
Trainer, 40-41
Transactional analysis, 79
Trust, 47, 183-184, 228

U

Ulschak, F. L., 62, 85, 154, 170, 194, 213
Unfreezing, 21-22, 191
University Associates, 250

V

Validity testing, 103
Values, 173-174, 229
Verbal communication, 194-195
Vincelette, J., 16

W

Weir, J., 31
Who, What, Why (WWW), 150
Windsor, R., 152